MILITARY AND VETERAN ISSUES

UNDERSTANDING MILITARY PERSONNEL AND RETURNING VETERANS

INFORMATION FOR SUBSTANCE USE TREATMENT PROVIDERS

MILITARY AND VETERAN ISSUES

Additional books in this series can be found on Nova's website under the Series tab.

Additional E-books in this series can be found on Nova's website under the E-book tab.

5

MILITARY AND VETERAN ISSUES

UNDERSTANDING MILITARY PERSONNEL AND RETURNING VETERANS

INFORMATION FOR SUBSTANCE USE TREATMENT PROVIDERS

AARON D. GOODMAN
EDITOR

NOVINKA

New York

For permission to use material from this book please contact us:
Telephone 631-231-7269; Fax 631-231-8175
Web Site: http://www.novapublishers.com

Library of Congress Cataloging-in-Publication Data

ISBN: 978-1-62808-636-2

Published by Nova Science Publishers, Inc. † New York

CONTENTS

Preface vii

Chapter 1 Addressing the Substance Use Disorder (SUD) Service Needs of Returning Veterans and Their Families: The Training Needs of State Alcohol and Other Drug Agencies and Providers 1
Kara Mandell, Marcia Trick, Jaclyn Sappah and Matthew Aumen

Chapter 2 Understanding the Military: The Institution, the Culture, and the People. Information for Behavioral Healthcare Specialists Working with Veterans and Service Members 59
Angela Halvorson

Index 97

PREFACE

Chapter 1 – The National Association of State Alcohol and Drug Abuse Directors (NASADAD) conducted an environmental scan of the training, outreach, and resources offered by the Single State Agencies (SSAs) in charge of drug and alcohol treatment and prevention services to respond to the needs of returning veterans and their families. This scan was conducted to learn how to more effectively serve returning veterans and family members impacted by substance use disorders (SUDs). To accomplish this, NASADAD conducted case studies of nine States that had been identified as having the largest number of initiatives for returning veterans. The data for these case studies were gleaned from 36 interviews with SSA staff and staff from publicly funded SUD treatment facilities. NASADAD staff gathered data on State policies, trainings, and outreach efforts, as well as recommendations for future development of technical assistance and training materials to address the gaps in services.

Specific requests to the States for technical assistance and trainings included:

- Trainings for substance use services providers, as well as primary care providers, to identify and treat post traumatic stress disorder (PTSD) and traumatic brain injury (TBI);
- Trainings on models to treat veteran-specific trauma;
- Trainings on military culture;
- Trainings to help law enforcement officials, the courts, and hospital workers identify veterans' SUDs; and
- Technical assistance to increase telehealth and webinar capabilities to overcome distance/ transportation barriers.

Chapter 2 – The U.S. Armed Forces are highly trained and ready to respond at a moment's notice to natural or human-made disasters anywhere in the country or the world. Yet many Americans' knowledge about the military is limited to what they have acquired from movies, books, and news reports. Few outside the military understand the culture, the values, or the people who make up the most powerful military force on earth.

What do people see in the U.S. Armed Forces that makes them dedicate their lives, and their families' lives, to military service? What is the U.S. military and who are the people who fill its ranks? How have the wars in Iraq and Afghanistan affected today's Armed Forces? What does this mean for the helping professionals who would serve them after they return from deployment?

This paper is designed to answer some of these questions by providing an overview of the military as an institution, the service members and their families who are the backbone of the institution, and how current military conflicts have affected service members, their families, and the future of military service.

The information contained herein is not an exhaustive overview of military culture but provides civilians, specifically behavioral healthcare specialists working with military personnel, with a basic understanding of the unique life and culture that is the military.

In: Understanding Military Personnel … ISBN: 978-1-62808-636-2
Editor: Aaron D. Goodman

Chapter 1

ADDRESSING THE SUBSTANCE USE DISORDER (SUD) SERVICE NEEDS OF RETURNING VETERANS AND THEIR FAMILIES: THE TRAINING NEEDS OF STATE ALCOHOL AND OTHER DRUG AGENCIES AND PROVIDERS*

Kara Mandell, Marcia Trick, Jaclyn Sappah and Matthew Aumen

EXECUTIVE SUMMARY

The National Association of State Alcohol and Drug Abuse Directors (NASADAD) conducted an environmental scan of the training, outreach, and resources offered by the Single State Agencies (SSAs) in charge of drug and alcohol treatment and prevention services to respond to the needs of returning veterans and their families. This scan was conducted to learn how to more effectively serve returning veterans and family members impacted by substance use disorders (SUDs). To accomplish this, NASADAD conducted

* This is an edited, reformatted and augmented version of the Substance Abuse and Mental Health Services Administration's Center for Substance Abuse Treatment, under the Partners for Recovery Initiative, dated September 2009.

case studies of nine States that had been identified as having the largest number of initiatives for returning veterans. The data for these case studies were gleaned from 36 interviews with SSA staff and staff from publicly funded SUD treatment facilities. NASADAD staff gathered data on State policies, trainings, and outreach efforts, as well as recommendations for future development of technical assistance and training materials to address the gaps in services.

Specific requests to the States for technical assistance and trainings included:

- Trainings for substance use services providers, as well as primary care providers, to identify and treat post traumatic stress disorder (PTSD) and traumatic brain injury (TBI);
- Trainings on models to treat veteran-specific trauma;
- Trainings on military culture;
- Trainings to help law enforcement officials, the courts, and hospital workers identify veterans' SUDs; and
- Technical assistance to increase telehealth and webinar capabilities to overcome distance/ transportation barriers.

INTRODUCTION

Over 1.6 million soldiers have been in theater in Afghanistan or Iraq since 2001. The pace of the deployments in these current conflicts is faster, deployments have been longer, and redeployment is more common than in the past (Tanielian et al., 2008). Repeated and extended deployments have been associated with increased SUDs and other health concerns (Eggleston, Straits-Trotter, and Kudler, 2009). In addition, recent studies (Hoge et al., 2004; Jacobson et al., 2008; Seal et al., 2009) have shown that veterans who experienced combat or other traumatic situations are at significantly elevated risk of SUDs, both pre- and postdischarge from service. Moreover, SUD symptoms can present years after discharge. Though all States (and their providers) have worked with veterans and their families since the 1970s or before, as more is learned about the unique substance use services needs of returning veterans, and as the SSAs and publicly funded SUD treatment and prevention providers are increasingly called on to prepare for and deliver substance use services for Operation Enduring Freedom and Operation Iraqi Freedom (OEF/OIF) veterans,[1] the States and SAMHSA have recognized that it is necessary to develop and identify specific strategies to address the substance use services needs of these veterans and their families.

The ***Partners for Recovery Initiative*** (under the Center for Substance Abuse Treatment [CSAT]) is interested in exploring the training needs of State alcohol and other drug agencies and the community-based prevention, treatment, and recovery support providers to ensure that the workforce is prepared to serve veterans. As a first step in this process, NASADAD conducted a preliminary environmental scan of selected States to learn about what specific kinds of trainings and outreach are being offered by the SSAs in charge of drug and alcohol treatment and prevention services in each State, and what trainings and technical assistance the States would like to receive. The results of that scan are presented in this document.

In July 2008, NASADAD queried its members about the SUD services that they provided for OEF/OIF veterans and their families. ***This brief inquiry*** asked States whether they had enacted 18 policies, services, and collaborations relationships that States have used to better serve OEF/OIF veterans and their families. NASADAD received responses from 45 States, representing 94 percent of the U.S. population.

NASADAD found there is great variation in the amount of activity that States are involved in when addressing the SUD needs of OEF/OIF returning veterans and their families. Many State agencies have already begun initiatives to address the SUD needs of these veterans, while others are only beginning to develop and implement plans.

Specifically, NASADAD learned that over half of the States have started critical interagency coordination with the U.S. Department of Veterans Affairs (VA), and the National Guard—but only eight have collaborated with the Department of Defense (DoD)/TRICARE. In addition, many States have basic policies in place to respond to the needs of veterans. In 31 States, SUD treatment providers are required to screen for veteran status; in 40 States, providers conduct screening to determine if clients need mental health assessments; and in 23 States, providers are required to screen for TBI. In addition, States have, at relatively low cost, delivered training on the unique needs of OEF/OIF veterans to SUD providers and counselors (13 States), provided information to SUD providers and counselors on services for veterans (22 States), and performed outreach and advertising to reach OEF/OIF veterans (16 States). However, NASADAD's July 2008 inquiry only revealed which types of strategies SSAs have implemented. It could not examine what they are doing in detail, or the effectiveness of any of the strategies that are being used in the States.

Methodology

Based on the results of the 2008 brief inquiry, nine States that reported the greatest activity targeted to veterans were chosen for the case studies. The nine States that participated in this study were Connecticut, New Mexico, New York, North Carolina, Oregon, Pennsylvania, Rhode Island, Utah, and Wyoming. States that have been particularly active in enacting policies and services and in collaborating with veterans' organizations provide rich information about their own and their providers' training needs. To collect the data for the report, NASADAD interviewed between two and six stakeholders who work at the State, local, or provider levels in each identified State. Interviews were conducted over the phone and lasted for approximately 1 hour, with followup questions answered via email.

A discussion guide was developed before interviews were conducted. Discussions were aimed to assess what interviewees perceived to be the most important training needs, *what* initiatives have been implemented or developed (especially training), and *how* these initiatives have been implemented at the policy and provider levels. Specifically, the topics for the interview included perceived need(s) for training, the kinds of initiatives that the interviewees participate in, the impetus for the initiatives, how the initiatives were envisioned and implemented, how the initiative is funded, any barriers that were encountered and how they were overcome, and how/if the effectiveness of the initiative is measured (i.e., outcomes). The discussion guide was reviewed by the NASADAD Research Committee, which is responsible for providing input on and approving proposed NASADAD inquiries. The guide is included in Appendix B of this document.

To complement the case studies, NASADAD acquired copies of curricula from trainings and other resources that have already been developed. NASADAD worked with the States to identify other OEF/OIF veteran-specific resources that may be helpful to other States and providers, including specific screening and assessment tools as well as treatment protocols. These documents are included in Appendix C.

Data Trends

To explore trends in the number of veterans who sought admission to the publicly funded treatment systems, NASADAD tabulated data from the Treatment Episode Data Set (TEDS; see Appendix A), which tracks information about admissions to publicly supported addiction treatment facilities. Though the scope of admissions included in TEDS is affected by differences in State reporting practices and varying definitions of treatment admission, TEDS primarily includes facilities that are licensed or certified by the State alcohol and drug agency, facilities that are funded by the SSA, and/or facilities that are required by State legislation to provide TEDS client-level data. Therefore, TEDS does not include all admissions to addiction treatment. A major population missing from TEDS data includes admissions to VA hospitals and facilities. In addition, not all States collect data on veteran status. Between 2000 and 2007, 32 States reported data continuously on veteran status. During this time period, 45 States reported data for at least 1 year. Trends in the data from the 45 States that reported data for at least 1 year are the same as trends in the 32 States that reported data continuously during this time period. Therefore, the following analyses use data from all 45 States that reported data.

The most significant finding was that only an average of 72,326 veterans admissions per year were reported in TEDS from 2000 to 2007 (the most recent year for which data are available). The actual number of admissions has ranged from 59,994 admissions in 2003 to 89,824 admissions in 2005. Figure 1 shows the total number of veterans admissions to substance use (SU) treatment across age groups reported to TEDS.

These admissions represent only a small proportion of veterans who are being treated for SUDs. This may be due to a variety of factors, including that veterans are not being treated in the publicly funded treatment system (i.e., they are being treated in VA facilities or privately funded facilities, which are not included in the TEDS universe) or a reluctance on the part of veterans to self-identify as an individual with a substance use disorder.

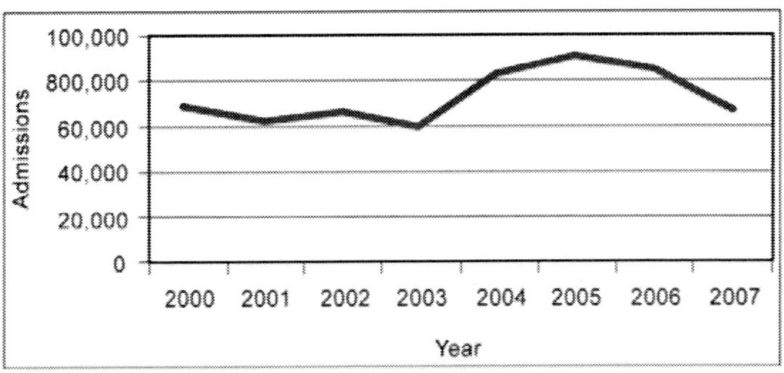

Figure 1. Total Veteran's Admissions to SU Treatment, 2000 – 2007.

Despite the relatively small number of veterans reported in the publicly funded systems, it is important to note that the total number of 18- to 29-year-old veterans (the veterans who most likely served in Iraq and Afghanistan during OEF/OIF), increased by 120 percent between 2000 and 2006. The number of 18- to 29- year- old veterans fell sharply in 2007, but remained 30 percent higher than the number of admissions for this group in 2000. This trend warrants further exploration. Figure 2 shows the number of veterans admissions to SU treatment reported to TEDS by age groups.

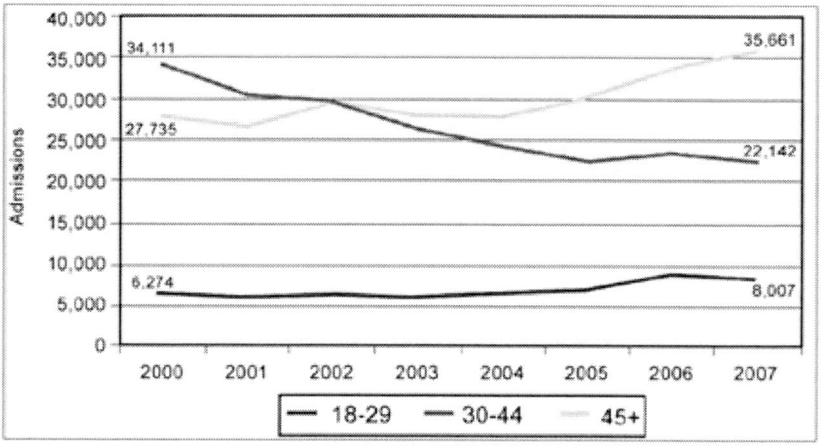

Figure 2. Veterans Admissions to SA Treatment by Age Group, 2000 -2007.

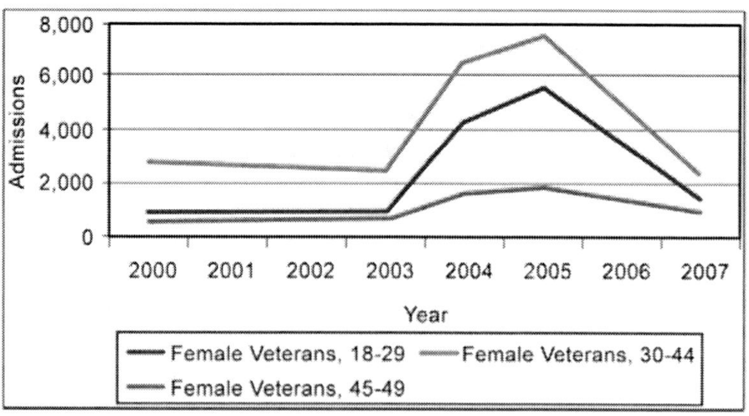

Figure 3. Admissions of Female Veterans to SA Treatment, 2000 – 2007.

Generally, women represent only about 10 percent of all veterans admissions captured in TEDS between 2000 and 2007. Nationally, the number of woman veterans admitted to the publicly funded substance use treatment system rose drastically in 2004 and 2005, and subsequently dropped equally as drastically in 2006 and 2007, particularly among woman veterans ages 18–44. During these dramatic increases, female veterans admissions rose to nearly 18 percent of all veterans admissions. This trend calls for additional research. Figure 3 shows the rise and fall of the numbers of women's admissions to treatment from 2000 through 2007.

The Substance Abuse and Mental Health Services Administration's (SAMHSA's) National Survey on Drug Use and Health (NSDUH) asks respondents: "Are you currently on active duty in the armed forces, in a reserves component, or now separated or retired from either reserves or active duty?" Combined data from the 2004–2006 NSDUH showed that one-quarter of veterans age 25 and under had suffered from SUDs in the preceding year, though it is impossible to discern from the NSDUH data whether these veterans had been deployed to combat zones. Unfortunately, the numbers of NSDUH respondents who self-identified as veterans in any given year (e.g., in 2007, 168 respondents reported being on active duty in the armed forces or in a reserves component, and 2,168 reported being separated or retired from either reserves or active duty) are too low to discern meaningful longitudinal trends. Finally, NSDUH cannot identify veterans who might have sought or did seek treatment.

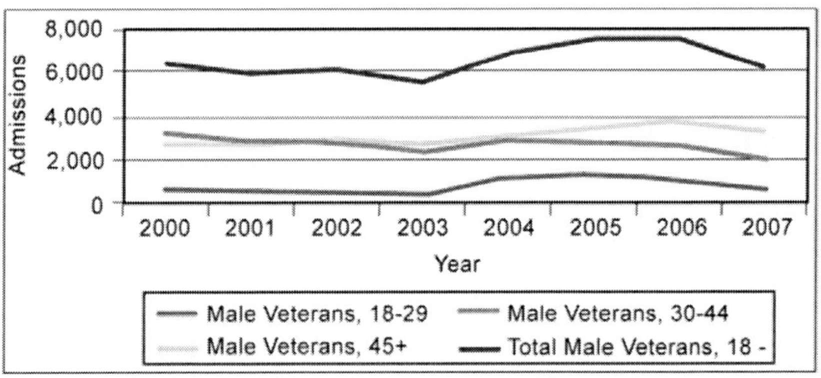

Figure 4. Male Veterans Admissions to SA Treatment, 2000 - 2007.

To better understand the data trends from TEDS, and to ascertain how the States are assisting their providers to better serve the SUD needs of returning veterans and their families, NASADAD staff conducted qualitative case studies of nine States. The nine States chosen for the case studies were those that had reported engaging in the largest number of initiatives focused on serving the SUD needs of veterans and their families. By documenting these efforts, other States can benefit from the lessons learned and resources that have been developed from other States.

A similar trend can be noted among male veterans admissions during the same time period, but the rise and fall of admissions is not nearly as drastic, as can be seen in Figure 4.

CASE STUDIES

These nine case studies provide a qualitative picture of the perceived training needs of SUD providers to address the unique needs of returning veterans and their families. To complete these case studies, NASADAD staff interviewed between two and six key stakeholders from each State, including the SSA; the National Treatment Network (NTN) representative; training or continuing education units (CEUs) staff; the staff responsible for veterans services in the SSA's office (if so designated); and providers identified by the SSA's office who participated in initiatives serving returning veterans and/or their families. Topics discussed included policy initiatives, trainings for providers, outreach initiatives, funding streams, and data collection.

Connecticut

The ***Connecticut Department of Mental Health and Addiction Services (DMHAS)*** is a combined mental health and addiction services agency. The Director of Veterans Services within DMHAS, Jim Tackett, oversees DMHAS's many veterans' initiatives.

DMHAS contracts with an administrative services agency, ***Advanced Behavioral Health***, to assist in recruiting, training, credentialing, and managing a statewide panel of licensed clinicians (private practitioners) interested in working with military personnel and their family members. To date, there are 235 licensed clinicians in the panel, which is accessed through a 24/7 call center. After a quick triage, the caller is provided the names of three clinicians in his or her neighborhood, and community case managers follow up on these calls to make sure that every caller is connected to services.

DMHAS staff believed that the overall barrier for veterans was access to care, so DMHAS recently enacted a new policy which mandates that veterans get the "next available bed" in their two residential substance use rehabilitation programs. Connecticut has found that automatically referring veterans to the VA without engaging them is often ineffective. They are addressing this issue by training providers on veterans issues and on the services that are available throughout the different systems. In addition, clinicians are encouraged to work with their VA counterparts to conduct discharge planning to assist veterans with their transition back to the community. Finally, regional DMHAS staff can evaluate whether veterans are eligible for VA care and if they meet DMHSAS eligibility requirements (unemployed, homeless). If veterans are eligible for both VA and DMHSAS services, they are given a choice.

The State of Connecticut is one of six States selected by SAMHSA to participate in a $2 million, 5-year ***Jail Diversion Program*** for veterans which involves a comprehensive strategic planning process and a pilot project in the Norwich/New London area. Four workgroups have been created: Benefits and Advocacy; Traumatic Brain Injury; Psycho-Social Supports; and Trauma-Integrated Care. A State advisory panel will resolve policy issues and also address sustainability issues. A local panel will provide aggressive outreach and training.

In 2004, the General Assembly appropriated $900,000 for the ***Military Support Program*** (MSP). The MSP became operational in March 2007; it instructed the State to provide outpatient behavioral health services to National Guard soldiers and their family members. The CT General Assembly has considered expanding the MSP beyond the reserves and their family members.

DMHAS collects data on all clients admitted to programs that receive State funding (including the MSP). Veteran status is established at intake, and DMHAS serves approximately 5,500 veterans a year. They are unaware, however, of how many OEF/OIF veterans are actually admitted into the system; DMHAS staff hopes to address this issue in the future.

In April 2008, DMHAS began to offer the Veterans Resource Representative Program—a 2-day training directed at DMHAS clinicians (see Appendix C for training handbook). In this program, key clinicians from the VA are brought in to talk about their programs covering such topics as eligibility criteria, enrollment processes, referral protocols, disability compensation, pension, home loan guarantee, and education benefits for veterans. A clinician from the PTSD anxiety clinic provides an overview of the clinical presentation of the newest generation coming home. Another expert on TBI discusses the difficulty in teasing out the differences between symptoms of PTSD and TBI. Clinicians receive 12 CEUs for attending the training. Seventy-five clinicians have been trained so far, but because of monetary restrictions DMHAS is unable to do the trainings more frequently than twice a year. The training is advertised in the DMHAS course catalog, and DMHAS did targeted outreach to encourage participation. Three of these trainings were conducted in 2008 and the first half of 2009; another is planned for October 2009.

The addiction treatment providers interviewed who had received the trainings rated them very highly, both clinically and in terms of education about systems, and expressed interest in attending other trainings. One provider suggested that, in lieu of receiving additional trainings, follow-up regional, quarterly meetings or calls to discuss lessons learned would be very useful. Another provider agreed, but thought that DMHAS specific trainings focusing only on addressing veterans issues within treatment centers would be helpful.

In addition, DMHAS organized two 2-day trainings conducted by the National Guard for their clinicians in the MSP in 2007; each clinician received 2 days of training and 6 CEUs per training day (12 CEUs in all). The panel members went through "Military 101" training (military organizational structure, policies, and procedures), and a clinician from the VA, Dr. Steven Southwick, provided training on new clinical thinking regarding PTSD. Topics of discussion included State VA benefits, TBI, and treatment modalities for PTSD (including Cognitive Processing Therapy), and DMHAS provided a detailed overview of the MSP. About 20 clinicians have joined the panel since then, and they have been trained individually.

To conduct outreach, Jim Tackett and his VA counterpart have given about 40 presentations across the State—to employers and teachers—to alert them to predictable symptoms of returning veterans and to encourage them to develop local programs. A summary report of the MSP, called "Findings on the Aftereffects of Service in Operations Enduring Freedom and Iraqi Freedom and The First 18 Months Performance of the Military Support Program," has also been completed (see Appendix C) and is being publicized (the 2004 legislation that authorized the MSP earmarked $500,000 for research). The local panel of the Jail Diversion Program will be providing educational activities in the pilot area for veterans who are at risk for arrest as well as for police officers during roll call and during a week- long crisis intervention training.

Beginning in April 2009, DMHAS received funding from the MSP to train and embed clinicians with Guard units that have been deployed or are soon to be deployed. Twenty-four Behavioral Health Advocates have been assigned to Guard units (14 are already embedded); they will participate in drill weekends with the unit (reimbursed for 4 hours)—either doing individual counseling or running workshops, depending on the psycho-education needs of the unit. The assigned clinician will act as the primary point of contact for National Guard members. When the unit deploys, the clinician will shift focus to the family members, and then will work with the unit when it returns. The clinician will provide the necessary services, but if the National Guard or family member needs services in another geographic area or another specialty, the clinician will refer to another MSP clinician. The clinicians will assist with the Yellow Ribbon Reintegration Program, a 30-day and 60-day prevention program aimed at reservists and their family members (a National Guard requirement introduced in March 2008 in a Defense Reauthorization Act). Jim Tackett has also provided outreach to the State Troopers Offering Peer Support (STOPS), as the State troopers have realized that many in their ranks are in the National Guard.

To complete this summary NASADAD staff talked to Jim Tackett, Director of Veterans Services; Marla Ackerley, Connecticut Valley Hospital–Merritt Hall; and Celeste Cremin-Endes, Director of Rehabilitation Services for Connecticut's Southwest Region.

New Mexico

The ***New Mexico Behavioral Health Collaborative*** oversees systems of care, data management, and performance and outcome indicators; monitors training; and funds both substance use and mental health services in the State of New Mexico. The Collaborative is unique in that it is a cabinet-level office representing 15 State agencies and the Governor's office.

In October 2007, the Collaborative began a pilot program in Sandoval County called ***Veteran and Family Support Services*** (VFSS). The VFSS initiative is a legislatively funded program focusing on providing triage, case management, and behavioral health services to veterans, service members, and their families, as needed. This initiative has targeted all veterans and their families, including veterans who are eligible for VA benefits, regardless of their ability to pay or their insurance status in the county. In addition to the pilot study, the collaborative maintains and staffs a dedicated telehealth connection room within the National Guard headquarters. This allows VFSS staff to provide brief interventions, triage services, and referrals to National Guard members who are not able to physically go to the VA facility. A VFSS program description and pamphlet are included in Appendix C. Collaborative staff have also agreed to begin a pilot program that will use Access to Recovery (ATR) vouchers to provide wraparound services for National Guard members. The ATR project is funded through a SAMHSA grant.

The VFSS project was funded by the New Mexico Legislature in 2006. In 2008, as a result of a request from Governor Richardson, the legislature provided VFSS with an additional $1.5 million to expand the VFSS project, specifically with regard to PTSD screenings and treatment.

In implementing the VFSS system, Collaborative staff emphasized the importance of family-centered treatment. An evaluation of the project showed that working with families led to positive outcomes. Veterans systems currently do not provide treatment to the families of veterans. In addition, transportation is a major barrier for veterans and their families in need of services. New Mexico has a large population of homeless veterans who are unable to get transportation to care centers, but even veterans who are not homeless can be hesitant to travel to receive services. The current telehealth services that the Collaborative offers are not sufficient to provide comprehensive services to all of New Mexico's veterans. The Collaborative is also working to diminish the stigma associated with having a mental health or substance use diagnosis, and to allow veterans and their families to maintain anonymity if desired, because it recognizes that there can be negative consequences to such diagnoses. Collaborative staff are working to create policies and practices that will allow veterans and their families to get help without being disempowered; they encourage policymakers to be supportive without labeling.

Minimal information is tracked on veterans and their families. Treatment providers collect veteran status at admission for the TEDS database, and VFSS staff have been working to develop strategies for more consistent data collection. They track direct services that are provided to returning veterans and their families, as well as individuals who were enrolled in direct service. Through the ATR pilot program, the collaborative will be able to track exactly what services veterans and their families are accessing.

All of the Collaborative's initiatives for returning veterans and their families are evaluated on an ongoing basis by staff at the University of New

Mexico, Deborah Altshul and Brian Isakson. Their evaluation of the VFSS initiative is included in Appendix C. Specifically the evaluators track the numbers of services provided, individual outcomes, and consumer satisfaction.

The Collaborative has just begun working to identify trainings on addressing the substance use needs of returning veterans and their families. At the December 2008 Behavioral Health Collaborative Conference, a speaker from the VA gave an overview about how to build DoD, VA, and community partnerships to support returning veterans and their families. The Collaborative has not determined if providers have all the skills necessary to serve the needs of returning veterans and their families. They hope to identify training needs through the ATR pilot study.

As part of its VFSS initiative, Collaborative staff have conducted extensive outreach to returning veterans and their families, military and veterans' advocacy groups, the courts and other social service providers to encourage these groups to refer their members and clients to VFSS services. VFSS has also participated in New Mexico's Yellow Ribbon weekends, making presentations to National Guard members and their families. Two additional counties not involved in the VFSS project, which have high proportions of veterans, have given out flashlights and other gadgets with a substance use hotline number (1-877-929-9797) on them to encourage veterans and their families to utilize this resource as a starting point for receiving SUD services.

To complete this summary NASADAD staff talked to Linda Roebuck, CEO, New Mexico Behavioral Health Collaborative/SSA; Harrison Kinney, New Mexico Behavioral Health Collaborative/NTN; Deborah Altshul, Primary Evaluator, University of New Mexico; and Chris Burmeister, VFSS.

New York

The ***Office of Alcoholism and Substance Abuse Services*** (OASAS) plans, develops, and regulates the public prevention and treatment system in New York State (NYS). OASAS staff conduct trainings for providers; license, fund, and supervise providers; and monitor substance use and use trends in the State. Though OASAS funds and supervises ***Samaritan Village***, which has had specific programs to address the substance use treatment needs of returning veterans since 1996, their involvement with returning veterans and their families has escalated in the past 2 years, beginning with their participation in ***SAM HSA's National Behavioral Health Conference and Policy Academy***

on Returning Veterans and their Families in August 2008. Since this meeting, the NYS agencies that participated in the Policy Academy continue to work together and meet monthly. OASAS also participates in the NYS Council on Returning Veterans and Their Families, a gubernatorial initiative, with several other State agencies and consumer representatives; the council meets quarterly. Both the Policy Academy Team and the council are targeting all veterans (regardless of discharge status), National Guard members, and family members of veterans. OASAS staff emphasize the importance of working with family members of veterans, a population that they believe is gravely underserved.

New York has several initiatives specifically to address the substance use treatment and prevention needs of returning veterans and their families. In 2008, four providers (including Samaritan Village) were selected for capital project awards to create 100 new residential beds specifically for returning veterans using one-time funding from legislative general funds. The State also allocated $280,000 for prevention counseling in schools near the Fort Drum base. OASAS has also identified two staff members as the designated leads to coordinate regional outreach and services specifically for returning veterans and their families in the upstate and downstate field offices. OASAS also conducts direct outreach at reunification weekends for returning National Guard members and their families, recruits veterans to work in the NYS substance use service system, and is in the process of planning three 90-minute trainings on returning veterans for their providers.

OASAS staff have identified two major barriers to creating initiatives for, and providing services to, returning veterans. Funding is the most significant barrier to addressing the needs of returning veterans and their families. State budgets are stretched thin and there are very few funds to start new programs or provide new trainings. Although OASAS had developed an "Action Plan" (see Appendix C) after participating in SAMHSA's Policy Academy on Returning Veterans and their Families, no funding was provided to finance the plan. In addition, OASAS staff believe that TRICARE is a barrier to access to substance use services for returning veterans and their families. TRICARE pays medical staff other than physicians (individual practitioners and organized providers) a very low rate for services and does not cover substance use services to the family members of returning veterans. Roy Kearse, Vice President of Samaritan Village, pointed out that most of the veterans that are treated by his agency have never been eligible for TRICARE benefits, either because they received a dishonorable discharge (possibly for using illicit drugs or alcohol), or because they are National Guard members.

Based on data from the NYS OASAS Data Warehouse, OASAS estimates that veterans represented 5 percent of all admissions in NYS from October 1, 2006 to September 30, 2007. During that year, there were 13,950 veteran admissions. More information on these admissions is included in the "Veteran Fast Facts" document in Appendix C. However, OASAS staff believe that this number is a significant undercount of the accurate numbers of veterans served. Beginning in 2009, all of the partner agencies involved in the NYS Council on Returning Veterans and Their Families identify veterans in the same way, by asking "have you served in the military?" This is important because people with less than honorable discharges and active-duty military are more likely to identify themselves this way. OASAS staff believe that even using this more global question, they will still be undercounting the number of veterans in the New York public substance use treatment system. In 2009, OASAS and its partner agencies are trying to identify and implement a similar question to be used across agencies to identify the family members of those who have served.

New York has two training mechanisms for its providers: OASAS conducts its own trainings and also certifies individuals and organizations to provide CEUs to providers in New York. OASAS delivers trainings via its online ***Addiction Medicine Free Educational Series***, which are workbooks about specific topics; individuals receive 1 CEU for each completed course in this series. To date, New York has only done one session of its Addiction Medicine series on ***identifying and working with clients who have TBI*** (see Appendix C). OASAS also presents biweekly, 90- minute webinars designed to enhance the skills and knowledge of the addiction profession in their ***Learning Thursdays*** initiative. Currently, Learning Thursdays trainings reach 400 substance use providers. These trainings are funded as part of OASAS's annual budget. OASAS training staff are currently developing the following webinars for the Learning Thursdays series: TBI Strategies (how to treat the substance use disorders of clients with TBI); Military 101 (an introduction to military culture); and TBI and Substance Abuse (the causal links between TBI and substance use). These topics were identified by the OASAS Training Division in March 2009, and the trainings were developed in May 2009. OASAS staff noted that online trainings are particularly effective for their providers because they can be accessed remotely and do not require providers to travel to a site-based training.

In addition to OASAS's trainings, several national and State-based training providers have been certified by OASAS to conduct trainings on the needs of returning veterans for providers in NYS (see "Learning and Development Initiatives for Addiction Providers Working With Veterans" in

Appendix C for examples of these trainings). In addition, the Institute for Professional Development in the Addictions, which serves as the New York Office of the Northeast Addiction Technology Transfer Center, has offered a series of free workshops on the needs of returning veterans, as well as quarterly returning veterans roundtables (see Appendix C for Veterans Roundtable agenda and presentations).

OASAS is confident that its providers are able to meet the SUD needs of OEF/OIF veterans. However, OASAS staff believe that providers need training on recognizing, treating, and referring patients with TBI and PTSD. Roy Kearse and Carol Davidson of Samaritan Village reemphasized the importance of cultural competency when working with returning veterans (they believe that most providers who are not returning veterans themselves have very little knowledge about the culture of the military), as well as the importance of helping veterans learn to secure safe housing. Lack of funding has prevented OASAS from conducting additional trainings.

The NYS Council on Returning Veterans and Their Families has adopted a “no wrong door” approach, and in support of that approach, each of the member agencies has been making presentations and providing updates to the other agencies to make them aware of what each agency is doing for returning veterans and their families. OASAS has also done outreach to providers in neighborhood health centers to teach them to make referrals to substance use providers. Finally, OASAS presents information about its initiatives for veterans and their families to substance use treatment and prevention providers during OASAS regional provider meetings.

OASAS conducts outreach with veterans and their families directly during reintegration weekends for National Guard members who are being released from active duty. OASAS is also committed to recruiting veterans from all wars to work in substance use services facilities. In support of this initiative, a $200 waiver is provided to returning veterans to take New York’s Credentialed Alcoholism and Substance Abuse Counselor licensure test. OASAS staff are also conducting an inquiry of publicly funded outpatient providers in NYS to determine the number of veterans currently working in the system. Lack of funding has prevented OASAS from conducting additional outreach.

To complete this summary NASADAD staff talked to Reba Architzel, Director, Bureau of Special Programs Financing, OASAS; Tom Nightingale, Associate Commissioner, Division of Treatment and Practice Innovation, OASAS; Paul Noonan, Training Coordinator, OASAS; Roy Kearse, Vice

President of Samaritan House; and Carol Davidson, Program Director of Samaritan Village's Veterans Program.

North Carolina

North Carolina has the fourth largest active-duty military population in the United States, distributed among eight military bases and 14 Coast Guard facilities. There are 110,000 active-duty soldiers and 25,000 reserve and National Guard soldiers employed in North Carolina. More than 792,000 veterans reside within the State, the 10th highest number in the country. There are over 3,000 reservists currently mobilized, and 35 percent of North Carolina's population is considered military, veteran, spouse, parent, or dependent.

The ***North Carolina Division of Mental Health, Developmental Disabilities and Substance Abuse Services*** (Division of MH/DD/SAS) leads the ***Governor's Focus on Returning Combat Veterans and Their Families task force***, an initiative mandated by the governor to "promote best practices in the service of veterans who served in the Global War on Terrorism and their families." The task force maintains a website, www.veteransfocus.org, which provides information about the prevalence of SUDs, mental health disorders, and TBI among veterans; a list of mental health, substance use, and TBI resources; resources for homeless veterans; and a toll-free information and referral telephone service for veterans called CARE-LINE, with trained staff answering calls 24 hours a day to answer questions, provide information, and make referrals. This website also provides a summary of, and the materials from, the 2006 Governor's Summit on Returning Combat Veterans and Their Families which endeavored to increase collaborations between Federal and State government, service providers, and programs to ensure the maximum level of care possible for OEF/OIF veterans (see Appendix C for more on the Governor's Summit). North Carolina also maintains the NCcareLINK website (www.nccarelink.gov), which lists information concerning programs and resources across the State and includes information specifically for military veterans. Veterans can access the site to locate the nearest center that provides services for their individual needs. In addition, upon return from deployment, informational packets and a letter from the Governor with a list of resources are also distributed to North Carolina veterans.

Data have been collected on veterans in North Carolina through the NC-Treatment Outcomes and Program Performance System (NC-TOPPS) as well as TEDS. The Governor's Focus on Returning Combat Veterans and Their Families website has minimal statistics available on veterans being served in the health care system. Currently, 12,000 North Carolina OEF/OIF veterans are enrolled with the Veterans Health Administration (VHA).

The Division of MH/DD/SAS has contracted with the North Carolina Area Health Education Centers (NC AHEC) Program to conduct training for service providers on the treatment needs of returning veterans and their families. "Painting a Moving Train," a presentation on PTSD and TBI, has educated 900 primary care providers and 350 substance use treatment professionals (see Appendix C for more information). NC AHEC hosts a podcast for the Citizen Soldier Support Program (CSSP) to present information on the mental health service needs of OEF/OIF veterans (see Appendix C for examples of podcasts). In addition, the Governor's Focus on Returning Combat Veterans and Their Families task force posts ***training opportunities*** on its website—including those from the University of North Carolina at Chapel Hill and NC AHEC (see Appendix C for examples of past trainings).

The Division of MH/DD/SAS staff noted that there are many barriers to conducting trainings for SUD providers. One potential obstacle centers on the ability to deliver the trainings that are available. It can be difficult for providers to travel to a central location for a workshop, and it can be costly to bring the workshop to the provider. Another need is for proper training in screening for specialty care, so that individuals who are not screened by their primary care physician do not go without needed services. There is also a desire to implement telehealth care in rural areas.

The Human Ecology Department at East Carolina University directs outreach services for veterans within the State. East Carolina University conducts one-on-one outreach to providers at no cost to the provider. The SSA also works in collaboration with the National Guard Drug Prevention Program, providers, and licensed treatment practitioners to provide assessments and referrals for service members identified with potential substance use disorders.

To complete this summary NASADAD staff talked to Flo Stein, SSA, North Carolina Division of MH/DD/SAS; Spencer Clark, NTN, North Carolina Division of MH/DD/SAS; John Harris, Veterans Mental Health Program Manager, North Carolina Division of MH/DD/SAS; and Barbara Davis, Director of Mental Health Education, Area L AHEC.

Oregon

In Oregon, the SSA is in a combined mental health/substance use department called the ***Addictions and Mental Health Division*** (AMH). Beginning in 2008, AMH has focused progressively more on the substance use and mental health services needs of returning veterans and their families. The Governor of Oregon, who is a veteran himself, established the ***Governor's Task Force on Veterans' Services***, and asked one of his advisors to focus specifically on veterans affairs in March 2008.

Although Oregon is not home to any military bases, it has the second largest number of deployed soldiers per capita in the nation. More than 7,000 National Guard men and women from Oregon have been deployed for active duty to Iraq and Afghanistan since September 11, 2001. The State will deploy another 3,000 National Guard members in May 2009. Services in Oregon continue to primarily target National Guard members and their families. The Governor's Task Force on Veterans' Services specifically examined the need for gender-specific services and focused on the special needs of woman veterans.

As Oregon continues to improve its services to returning veterans and their families, the task force is looking across the nation to identify best practices to better serve that population. They are specifically interested in learning about jail diversion programs, including veterans courts, and trainings for law enforcement officers about how to recognize and address veterans issues. In December 2008, the task force released ***a report*** (see Appendix C) detailing their findings and recommendations for improvements in a variety of areas, including mental health and addiction service delivery that affect the lives of veterans and their families. Although AMH currently is not systematically collecting any data, they have contracted with a consultant to do a stakeholder analysis. This analysis is being financed through AMH funding.

A policy action package, titled "Addiction Services for Uninsured Workers and Returning Veterans," was proposed by AMH for 2009–11 (see Appendix C for the full document). If AMH receives the $5,710,000 necessary for its implementation, the package will support "outreach, brief intervention services and outpatient addiction treatment to 3,000 workers and returning veterans who have substance use and/or co-occurring substance use and mental health disorders and are uninsured or have exhausted their healthcare benefits" (Department of Human Services, Policy Option Package 2009-2011).

Oregon's rural areas specifically face numerous challenges exacerbated by geography. For veterans and their families who live in rural areas, traveling to and from distantly located VA facilities becomes a major inconvenience as well as a financial burden that can ultimately prevent them from obtaining necessary addiction services. In addition, according to findings from the task force, existing access for addiction services in remote/rural areas of the State is insufficient for the current and projected needs of veterans and families. Finally, no residential or inpatient program exists in the VA system that allows children to accompany their mother into treatment, which is often a deterrent for women who might otherwise seek care.

AMH has recognized the need to create training programs for their providers on the needs of returning veterans and their families. Currently, they hold biannual meetings that provide training and presentations on the latest research for mental health/substance use providers, and they believe that this would be a good venue to provide such trainings (see "Working With Trauma Survivors in Appendix C for an example training). AMH staff are currently trying to identify trainings and trainers that would be appropriate for this conference.

The Governor's Task Force on Veterans' Services identified trauma as a major issue for returning veterans and their families, particularly military sexual trauma, which disproportionately affects women. There are no gender-specific VA treatment facilities in Oregon; this is a barrier for women, who are more comfortable and have better outcomes when they receive such treatment (e.g. child care and prenatal care). In addition, substance use providers' lack of knowledge about PTSD/TBI in working with returning veterans and their families is a major barrier found in Oregon's addiction treatment system. Identifying PTSD, TBI, and SUD continues to be a problem in Oregon, and AMH staff are working to identify appropriate screening and assessment tools.

AMH staff, in conjunction with other entities (including the Oregon National Guard), regularly conduct pre- and postdeployment outreach on substance use and mental health services to returning veterans and their families. This outreach includes a series of discussions, along with the appropriate referral information and resources for veterans and their families, by the Oregon National Guard Reintegration Team. AMH compiles a yearly State directory of providers that is shown to returning veterans and their families in a PowerPoint presentation. In addition, AMH uses the Reintegration Team's monthly newsletter as a publicity tool for its alcohol and drug use hotline.

The task force found that despite this outreach, veterans and their families still were unaware of many of the services that were available to them. To address this problem, they recommended the creation of a one-stop web-based

"Bulletin Board"–type resource to provide a clearinghouse of information for service members and their families.

To complete this summary NASADAD staff talked to Karen Wheeler, NTN/Addictions Policy Manager, and Diane Lia, Women's Services Network (WSN), from the Addictions and Mental Health Division and Elan Lambert, Director of National Alliance on Mental Illness (NAMI) Oregon, to learn about the ways Oregon has responded to the needs of OEF/OIF veterans.

Pennsylvania

The ***Pennsylvania Bureau of Drug and Alcohol Programs*** (BDAP) is charged with developing and implementing a comprehensive health, education, and rehabilitation program for the prevention, intervention, treatment, and case management of drug and alcohol use and dependence. This program is implemented through grant agreements with the 49 Single County Authorities (SCAs) who, in turn, contract with private service providers. Each of the SCAs operates independently and handles its own administrative oversight, funding, and program initiatives while BDAP provides for central planning, management, and monitoring. Programs are funded with State and Substance Abuse Prevention and Treatment Block Grant funds. The State only collects data on returning veterans through the TEDS systems.

Since 2005, BDAP has participated in the PA Returning Military Task Force, or PA CARES (www.pacares.org). This group meets monthly to address the various needs of Pennsylvania service members returning from Afghanistan and Iraq. The group was developed by Jane Bishop and Captain James Joppy and includes about 20 partners from various State departments, military veterans, advocacy associations, and others. BDAP ensures that a representative takes part in the monthly meetings.

In September 2007, the Pennsylvania Regional Drug and Alcohol Training Institute (developed by BDAP and implemented through ***the Institute for Research, Education and Training in Addictions*** [IRETA]) hosted a 3-day training titled ***"Serving T ho se Who Serve: Veterans and Their Families"*** (see Appendix C for the training agenda). The training was offered to the SCAs as well as to providers within the State. State dollars from BDAP's budget supported the training through the Department of Health. Topics included Treatment for Veterans with PTSD, Secondary Stress, and Addiction Issues; Issues That Impact Women in the Military; Addressing and Treating the Stressors on Families of the Veterans; Traumatic Brain Injury; and

Veterans and Homelessness. See Appendix C for Summary of Guidelines for Field Management of Combat-Related Head Trauma.

The State of Pennsylvania partners with IRETA, as well as with the ***Northeast Addiction Technologies Transfer Center*** (NeATTC) to provide trainings on various facets of SUD treatment and prevention, including serving returning veterans. As a complement to these trainings, IRETA hosts online newsletters developed by NeATTC to provide education and training for providers. CEUs are offered to those who read the newsletters. In 2002, a newsletter titled ***"Traum a, Terrorism , and Substance Abuse"*** focused on substance use and PTSD (see Appendix C).

Several training barriers persist within the State. Of prime importance are the financial barriers and the ability to bring providers to the trainings that are offered. Webinars are being utilized to conduct trainings for medical professionals, but they are not yet readily available for addiction issues. It was noted through the interview process that there is great expertise within the substance use system, but the system is underfunded and collaboration between the substance use field and the State Department of Veterans Affairs is lacking. Training for providers also needs to be ongoing. Providers must be aware of the latest research, treatment protocols, and needs of veterans.

Outreach activities are conducted by individual SCAs, independently of BDAP. One example provided of such activities within the State is an outreach van in Scranton that disseminates information to returning combat veterans. Pennsylvania also relies on its Vet Centers (free services provided to all combat veterans through the VA) and veteran advocacy organizations to conduct outreach services. Outreach services were, however, identified as a greater need throughout the interviews conducted.

To complete this summary NASADAD staff spoke with Jeffrey Geibel, Drug and Alcohol Program Supervisor, BDAP; William Noonan, Program Analyst, BDAP; Michael Flaherty, Executive Director, IRETA; and Jim Aiello, Director, NeATTC.

Rhode Island

The Rhode Island ***Department of Mental Health, Retardation, and Hospitals*** is responsible for providing access and support for those with substance use and mental health issues, as well as developmental disabilities. The ***Division of Behavioral Healthcare Services (DBH)*** within the department was very active in the ***Veterans Task Force*** from 2005 to 2008.

Due to budgetary restrictions, DBH employees have not participated in the task force over the last year, but they are hoping to reengage with this group in the future.

In 2005, the New England ATTC, which is based in Rhode Island, collaborated with DBH and various branches of the military and community organizations to create ***The Rhode Island Blueprint*** (see Appendix C), a document outlining strategic steps to create a system of care for returning veterans; this blueprint has been used as a model by the Department of Defense. More information about the Veterans Task Force, including the Blueprint, ***a draft handbook,*** and agendas of task force meetings, is available on their website, http://states.ng.mil/sites/RI/Resources/vettaskforce/default.aspx. This initiative resulted in the identification of a military liaison within the Rhode Island Family Court system, evening programs in both the primary health care clinic and the Addictions Treatment program at the VA Medical Center, and the development of a workforce training project with the Rhode Island Council of Community Mental Health Organizations.

Activities for veterans have, in the past, been paid for out of the DBH budget. Currently, DBH is using a SAMHSA grant to increase supportive housing for veterans and is applying for a SAMHSA Jail Diversion grant (5-year grant for close to $400,000 each year), to divert veterans and others with mental illness, such as trauma-related disorders, from the criminal justice system to community-based trauma-integrated services. DBH is considering using ATR money to provide vouchers to allow veterans to access assessments and case management.

At least two of Rhode Island's substance use providers have a contract with DoD/TRICARE to provide services for veterans. One of these providers offers clinical services that are provided by the VA, while substance use staff members arrange for transportation and the delivery of services. Despite these provider community based organizations and VA collaborations, DBH staff noted that most veterans served by their system do not have TRICARE health insurance and most mental health/substance use providers in Rhode Island are not part of the TRICARE network.

Currently, DBH collects information on veteran status on mental health patients only; addiction providers can report their clients' veteran status in TEDS at this time, but when the mental health and substance use systems merge this year, reporting veteran status will be required for substance use clients as well.

DBH has not provided recent trainings regarding the substance use service needs of returning veterans and their families. They, however, provide scholarships for the ***New England School of Addiction Studies***, where training is offered on PTSD and substance use.

Veterans Task Force committees have undertaken the bulk of the outreach activities for returning veterans in Rhode Island. They have set up a website for women veterans and have provided training for employers to better respond to needs of veterans (see Appendix C). They have also developed and broadcast public service announcements (PSAs) and television announcements. Finally, the task force conducts peer-to-peer training, which trains eight National Guard members and eight civilians to provide assistance to guardsmen. The eight National Guard members that are trained in this program are then embedded in units to help soldiers. If the veteran does not wish to go through the military channels for service, that person is referred to the civilian counterpart to provide referrals.

To complete this summary NASADAD staff interviewed Rebecca Boss, NTN, Corinna Roy, Behavioral Health Planner, and Lori Dorsey, WSN and Public Health Promotion Specialist from DBH; Kathy Rathbun, Director, NRI Community Services; Judy Bolzani, Director of Residential and Substance Abuse and Supported Housing Services at Wilson House; and Dr. Susan Storti, New England School of Addiction Studies.

Utah

There are a total of 16,000 veterans in Utah, and it is estimated that 13,000 Utah service members have been deployed during OEF/OIF. The ***Utah Division of Substance Abuse and Mental Health*** (DSAMH) is a combined substance use and mental health agency, working with counties that are authorized as 13 local authorities (10 of those local authorities are combined substance use and mental health). In its veterans initiatives to date, DSAMH has focused primarily on expanding mental health services. DSAMH has participated in monthly meetings of the Veterans and Families Counseling Committee (VFCC), which was convened by the Utah Legislature beginning in 2006, along with representatives of the National Guard, the Utah Veterans Administration, the Brain Injury Association of Utah, DoD, and veterans and family members, to address the needs of returning veterans and their families. Utah's efforts have been targeted at the families of veterans, because they believe that this is the best way to engage the veterans. They have also targeted active Utah National Guard members.

The Utah legislature passed the Counseling for Families of Veterans bill in 2006, which provided $210,000 for fiscal year (FY) 2007; $210,000 for FY 2008; $100,000 for FY 2009, and $50,000 for FY 2010 to address veterans' issues. Currently the Mental Health Services Division of DSAMH administers the VFCC's funds, but that responsibility will shift to the State Department of Veterans Affairs in July 2009. In addition to funding the VFCC, this expenditure has funded two surveys. The first survey queried providers about existing services for veterans and their families. From this survey, the VFCC concluded that Utah has sufficient capacity to serve veterans and their families with SUDs, but that veterans and their families were not utilizing the services that were available. The second survey was distributed to veterans and tried to identify the reason that they were not utilizing services. From this survey, VFCC members concluded that the reasons were (1) a lack of awareness of existing resources and (2) the stigma attached to using substance use and mental health services.

Utah's NTN representative, Dave Felt, reported that, anecdotally, Utah has seen no increase in utilization of addiction treatment services by veterans or increases in crisis calls. Bart Davis, the Transition Assistance Advisor for the Utah National Guard and Reserves, who helps National Guard members and reservists navigate DoD and VA services, has been able to link every veteran that has contacted him with appropriate services. DSAMH employees believe that most new veterans are utilizing benefits from the VA or private insurance rather than entering the publicly funded addiction system.

Since 2006, over 400 people have attended free trainings conducted by various branches of the military. The trainings focused on OEF/OIF readjustment issues and on recognizing and treating PTSD. One 2-hour session was aimed at mental health and addiction treatment professional counselors, church leaders, and city and county leaders; the session described clinical symptoms of PTSD and other signs to look for that might prompt referrals to services. The second 2-hour session was designed for veterans and their families and discussed, in more general terms, readjustment issues and symptoms of PTSD as well as information on how to obtain help, general veterans benefits, VA hospital and veterans center resources, and other topics. SUDs were mentioned briefly in these trainings but were not discussed in detail.

On April 1–2, 2009, DSAMH held its Generations Conference, an annual 2-day conference targeted at mental health providers (DSAMH's conference for addiction providers takes place in the fall); both public and private providers were invited, and about 500 people attended. A number of sessions were devoted to veterans' issues. The sessions included information on PTSD and TBI clinical considerations in treating veterans. The keynote speaker was Eric Newhouse (a specialist in PTSD and TBI). Eighty-five veterans and family members were invited to the conference for free.

In the future, DSAMH staff would like to develop a DVD to train law enforcement officers on effectively addressing in-home violence and diffusing hostage situations with returning veterans.

The state of Utah developed a DVD, "Benefits for all Utah Veterans," that encourages veterans and their family members to seek the wide range of services that are available to them, including services related to physical or emotional health issues, vocational services, and so on. The DVD was sent to all known family members of veterans (12,000) in all the different branches of the military. The DVD presents the Governor and the four commanders of the different branches of the Utah National Guard encouraging veterans to seek any services they might need. Rather than outlining all the services (telephone numbers and a link to their website, www.utvethelp.com are provided), the DVD attempts to dispel the mindset that the VA's services are only for those who are severely wounded and to encourage people to consider seeking help for their family member. A segment also addresses the myth that a PTSD diagnosis will automatically affect a security clearance, when in fact there has to be a defect in sound judgment and there is a low risk of a PTSD diagnosis affecting a security clearance.

DSAMH staff have learned that the timing of when to conduct outreach with returning veterans is important. Rather than overwhelming the returning veterans with prevention education materials immediately upon their return, it is more effective to give them a brief orientation upon their return and then wait 3–6 months to present the bulk of the material, when symptoms might be starting to appear and veterans and their families would be more receptive to the outreach. In the most recent VFCC meeting, it was noted that symptoms are appearing in about a year, and that this might be a good time to provide interventions and materials.

To complete this summary NASADAD staff interviewed David Felt, NTN, and Ron Stamberg, Director of Mental Health Services, DSAMH.

Wyoming

Although providers in Wyoming have been treating veterans for many years, the combined mental health/substance use department, the ***Mental***

Health and Substance Abuse Services Division (MHSASD) has undertaken various initiatives to systematically address the substance use and mental health services needs of returning veterans and their families since 2007. In 2007, MHSASD, in conjunction with the Wyoming Veterans Commission, formed a task force to assess and address the needs of returning veterans and their families. The group conducted a gaps analysis to identify several short-term and long-term needs that the Federal government is not currently addressing. The analysis also identified the resources and services necessary to fill these gaps (see The Wyoming Department of Health's "Executive Report on Veterans' Mental Health Needs" in Appendix C for more details).

During the gaps analysis, the task force found that providers' lack of knowledge regarding veteran resources/benefits and PTSD/TBI are the major barriers within the health care system. MHSASD hopes to obtain funding for housing and financial planning to help stabilize returning veterans and their families with mental health/substance use problems; this stability is necessary to allow returning veterans and their families to confront the source of their problems.

In addition to conducting trainings for providers and outreach to returning veterans and their families, MHSASD gives families a telephone number for MHSASD that they can call for help with almost anything—ranging from a broken refrigerator to an emergency contact for the brigade. Since the beginning of 2008, MHSASD has been transporting counselors, physicians, and psychiatrists to rural communities without VA medical facilities in order to provide OEF/OIF veterans and their families with needed care. MHSASD also reimburses OEF/OIF veterans and their families for mileage to travel to a VA facility from a rural community. MHSASD also provides reimbursement for veterans and their families to travel to a MHSASD funded services when they are not eligible for VA benefits.

The Wyoming State Legislature appropriated $848,000 in 2008 to address gaps in service identified by the task force. The funding allows for the contracted services of two Veterans Advocates whose duties include assisting soldiers and their families who may be in need of mental health or addiction treatment services. The appropriation also included $68,000 for reimbursement of physicians to provide assessments; $250,000 to reimburse soldiers and their families for such items as childcare, transportation, and mileage to access mental health or addiction treatment services; $40,000 to provide training to physicians and other health care providers on war-related injuries and illnesses; and $50,000 to provide reintegration training for community leaders and employers.

MHSASD informally tracks treatment services, including assessments, of OEF/OIF veterans visiting publicly funded providers only. In the opinion of Ronda Brauburger, the Veterans Advocate, OEF/OIF returning veterans are unique because society is now aware of and can look for the symptoms of PTSD and other mental health/substance use conditions when they return from combat. She believes that TBI is more prevalent within OEF/OIF veterans because of their increased exposure to explosions.

MHSASD uses the legislative appropriation to host a number of training programs with the objective of improving services for returning veterans and their families. Annually, they organize a statewide 2½-day training called "The Wounded Warrior Wellness Workshop: Preparing Professionals to Meet the Needs of Veterans" to prepare the community for the return of veterans. MHSASD uses this workshop as a mechanism to target the entire community, including primary care physicians, nurses, mental health/addictions providers, police officers, and families, regarding TBI, PTSD, and available resources from MHSASD and the Wyoming Department of Veterans Affairs. Although the workshop targets the community at large, it does have several tracks specific to mental health and addictions providers. They are planning on videotaping the Wounded Warrior Workshops and translating them into a series of three webinars for non-attendees to view. Attendees will receive CEUs for attending the workshop or participating in the webinar.

In November 2007 the Wyoming Department of Health, including MHSASD, partnered with the Wyoming Military Department to host an educational training conference at Camp Guernsey for Wyoming health providers and military leaders. The conference was designed to give attendees a more detailed background regarding war-related illnesses and injuries. The Wyoming Life Resource Center in Lander also offers assessment services and TBI training for providers working with veterans and their families.

A barrier identified by the State is that many primary care physicians do not attend these specialty trainings, for reasons such as a lack of awareness, funds, or desire, and they lack the training for assessing PTSD, TBI, and other SUDs. It is important for physicians to have a good understanding of the resources available to this population, but the vast distances between providers make it difficult for MHSASD to conduct statewide trainings. The integration of telehealth technology will be useful in overcoming this barrier.

MHSASD staff have conducted outreach to returning veterans and their families, as well as providers. The department participates in and provides resources to be handed out at the National Guard's Yellow Ribbon Program in Wyoming. MHSASD runs another program, similar to the Yellow Ribbon

Program, called the Family Readiness Fair. This event, which is held prior to deployment, focuses on the soldiers and their families, offering trainings in various problem areas (e.g., maintaining relationships while apart), resources for connecting with providers and other relevant assistance, and educational materials about maintaining healthy lives and looking for warning signs of conditions such as PTSD and TBI. Staff have also embarked on an advertising campaign to increase community awareness of the needs of returning veterans and their families. As part of this campaign, staff have spoken on radio shows, distributed written material throughout the State, and created informative websites.

Conducting outreach to primary care physicians to help them identify and refer patients with SUDs has been a priority for MHSASD. In 2007, MHSAD sent a letter, screening instrument, and referral information to primary care physicians throughout Wyoming. The task force also prompted Governor Freudenthal to mail a letter to the Wyoming Medical Society encouraging Wyoming primary health providers to become TRICARE providers.

MHSASD staff understand that support is necessary for providers to successfully conduct outreach efforts on behalf of veterans. They also believe that without outreach State initiatives will have a minimal impact.

To complete this summary NASADAD spoke with Rodger McDaniel, Deputy Director, Laura Griffith, Program Manager, Regina Dodson, Veterans Specialist and Ronda Brauburger, Veterans Advocate, of MHSASD to learn about the ways Wyoming has responded to the needs of OEF/OIF returning veterans.

FINDINGS

Below is a chart that summarizes target populations among service members and their families, a brief list of State-sponsored trainings for service providers, initiatives to assist veterans and their families, and outreach initiatives that have been undertaken by the SSA in each of the nine case study States. The chart also summarizes barriers identified by the SSA in each of the nine States.

	Target Population	Trainings for Providers	Initiatives for Veterans and Their Families	Outreach Initiatives	Barriers Identified
Connecticut	National Guard soldiers and their family members (Military Support Program [MSP]) Veterans at risk for arrest (Jail Diversion Program)	Veterans Resources Representative Training Program Trainings for MSP clinicians	"Next available bed" policy MSP Jail Diversion Program Embedded Behavioral Health Advocates	Conducted outreach to: State Troopers Offering Peer Support (STOPS) Employers and teachers Veterans and their families	Transportation Lack of data on the number of veterans/family members admitted into the system Access to care (not enough beds) Referrals without engagement Need for better coordination between the SSA and the VA
New Mexico	National Guard members All veterans and their families	General session on "Building Department of Defense, VA and Community Partnerships: Working to Support Veterans of Iraq and Afghanistan and their Families"	Veteran and Family Support Services (VFSS) Access to Recovery	Conducted outreach to returning veterans and their families, military and veterans' advocacy groups, the courts and other social services providers (VFSS) Handed out flashlights with the substance use hotline number in non-VFSS areas	Transportation Funding
New York	All veterans regardless of discharge status National Guard members	Web-based Trainings: TBI Strategies, TBI and Substance Abuse, Military 101	"No wrong door" approach Prevention counseling in schools	Conducted outreach during reunification weekends with National Guard members and their families	Transportation Funding TRICARE

	Target Population	Trainings for Providers	Initiatives for Veterans and Their Families	Outreach Initiatives	Barriers Identified
	Families of veterans	Partners with the Northeast Addiction Technology Transfer Center (NeATTC) to provide additional trainings		Conducted outreach to the other agencies participating in the NY State Council on Returning Veterans and their Families to make them more aware of resources	
North Carolina	Veterans who served in the Global War on Terrorism and their families	Regional and web-based trainings through the Area Health Education Centers (NC AHEC) Program	Web-based resource lists	Outreach conducted to individual providers on the needs of returning veterans and their families by East Carolina University	Transportation Funding
Oregon	National Guard members and their families Female veterans	Currently trying to identify trainings and trainers that would be appropriate	Proposed creation of a one-stop web- based information clearinghouse	Conducts outreach with the National Guard to National Guard members and their families Publicizes a list of providers and a substance use hotline number	Transportation Substance use providers' lack of knowledge about PTSD/TBI Identifying appropriate screening and assessment tools
					Lack of VA facilities that allow children to accompany their parents into SUD treatment Despite outreach, veterans and their families still unaware of many available services

(Continued)

	Target Population	Trainings for Providers	Initiatives for Veterans and Their Families	Outreach Initiatives	Barriers Identified
Pennsylvania	Identified by the Single County Authorities (SCAs)	Partnered with IRETA to host "Serving Those Who Serve: Veterans and Their Families" and publish web-based newsletters Department of Health trainings: Treatment for Veterans With PTSD, Secondary Stress and Addiction Issues; Issues That Impact Women in the Military; Addressing and Treating the Stressors on Families of the Veterans; Traumatic Brain Injury; Veterans and Homelessness	Conducted by the SCAs	Conducted by the SCAs Vet Centers and advocacy organizations PA cares website	Transportation Funding Need better collaboration between PA Bureau of Drug and Alcohol Programs (BDAP) and VA
Rhode Island	All veterans and their families	Work with New England School of Addition Studies to provide trainings	Supportive housing initiative	RI Veterans Task Force has:	Transportation Funding/staffing
	National Guard members Female veterans and National Guard members	Peer-to-peer training	Workforce training project with the Rhode Island Council of Community Mental Health Organizations Created a military liaison within the Family Court system	Created public service announcements Conducted outreach to employers Created a website for woman veterans	

	Target Population	Trainings for Providers	Initiatives for Veterans and Their Families	Outreach Initiatives	Barriers Identified
Utah	Families of veterans National Guard members	Generations Conference sessions on veterans issues	"Benefits for all Utah Veterans" DVD sent to all families	Outreach conducted when National Guard members return from combat and 3–6 months post return Distributes the DVD "Benefits for all Utah Veterans"	Transportation Lack of awareness of existing resources Stigma
Wyoming	National Guard members	"The Wounded Warrior Wellness Workshop: Preparing Professionals to Meet the Needs of Veterans" Wyoming Life Resource Center offers TBI training	Veterans Advocates Wyoming State Training School offers assessment services Provide transportation	Outreach to primary care physicians Participates in and provides resources to be handed out at the National Guard's Yellow Ribbon Program Family Readiness Fair Advertising campaign	Lack of knowledge regarding veteran resources/benefits and PTSD/TBI Funding for housing and financial planning Transportation/ distance between providers and clients

Note: IRETA = Institute for Research, Education, and Training in Addictions; PTSD = posttraumatic stress disorder; TBI = traumatic brain injury; VA = U.S. Department of Veteran Affairs.

THEMES

Though each State case study is unique, several themes became apparent upon analysis. These themes can be grouped in several topic areas: lack of data; targeted populations; need for training resources and evidence-based practices; common barriers and key issues. A summary and more extensive discussion of the themes are provided below. The themes provide valuable information for planning future services for veterans and their families.

Lack of Data

- Most States capture limited data on veterans and their family members.
- Data are often considered to be an underestimate of the numbers of veterans served in the substance use systems.
- Data are not captured consistently from State to State.
- Service data are not routinely tracked on veterans and family members between the substance use system and the VA system.

Targeted Populations

- All States provide services to veterans in combat and noncombat situations, dating back to World War II.
- Most States identified National Guard members as a priority population.
- Family members of veterans were identified by several States as target populations.

Need for Training Resources and Evidence-Based Practices

- States noted the need for information on evidence-based practices for returning veterans and their families, particularly for OEI/OIF veterans.
- States seek resources, such as screening and assessment tools.
- States require training and training materials, particularly on PTSD, TBI, and military culture.

Common Barriers

- Funding, particularly to expand services and to provide training
- Transportation
- Collaboration with and knowledge of the VA

Key Issues

- Strong leadership from the Governor, State funding, and cross-systems collaboration were key elements to the success of these State efforts targeted to addressing the substance use issues of returning veterans and their families.
- Three States emphasized the "no wrong door approach," which provides individuals easy access to services wherever they enter the system.
- Five States mentioned the importance of coordination, communication, and linkages between the SSA and the VA.
- Lastly, several States noted the importance of providing holistic services to veterans and their family members.

Lack of Data

The lack of accurate data on the number of veterans was frequently identified as an issue in States. Seven of the nine case study States can provide an estimate of the numbers of veterans in their systems. However, most believe that these numbers are significantly lower than the actual numbers of veterans served. Several States emphasized that the way questions are asked regarding veteran status led to undercounting. For example, many people who have served in the National Guard, or who have been less than honorably discharged, are not considered "veterans." Additionally, many veterans are hesitant to reveal their status because of stigma associated with addictions. Active military members may experience fear of negative repercussions, including effects on security clearances and promotions and the ability to redeploy.

In addition, because little is understood about the unique needs of OEF/OIF veterans and their families, or what trainings need to be provided to help substance use providers address these needs, it is important to track actual services that veterans are receiving. Connecticut found that many referrals to

VA treatment were not leading to engagement. New Mexico has begun to use electronic health records to track the referrals. Rhode Island is considering using the Access to Recovery voucher system to track services; New Mexico has already begun that process. No States are currently tracking access to SUD services by the families of veterans.

Targeted Populations

Each of the nine case study States provides addiction treatment services to veterans who served in a variety of combat and noncombat situations, including veterans who served during World War II, as well as active members of the military and their families. All of the States have targeted what they perceive as underserved populations of veterans and their families. In seven of the nine States (Connecticut, New Mexico, New York, Oregon, Rhode Island, Utah, and Wyoming), the SSA has identified National Guard members as a priority population. Their rationale for this is that National Guard members have access to fewer benefits and services, and often received less preparation prior to deployment. Seven of the nine States (Connecticut, New Mexico, New York, North Carolina, Oregon, Rhode Island, and Utah) have also identified the families of veterans as another targeted population. These States explained that they believe that families of veterans are underserved, and often are the first to ask for help when a veteran experiences the symptoms of PTSD, TBI, or an SUD. Through its SAMHSA-funded Jail Diversion Program, Connecticut has been able to target veterans at risk of arrest. Because of the large numbers of recently discharged veterans in North Carolina, the SSA in that State has focused specifically on serving veterans who served in the war on terrorism and their families. In Oregon, female veterans are another targeted population because of perceived additional barriers to treatment, including the lack of VA facilities that allow children to accompany their parents into SUD treatment, and because of the prevalence of military sexual trauma, which often leads to SUDs and disproportionately affects women.

Need for Training Resources and Evidence-Based Practices

From these case studies, NASADAD learned that initiatives directed at addressing the substance use needs of returning veterans and their families are new and varied. Many States noted difficulty in identifying evidence-based practices for serving returning veterans and their families with SUDs, particularly for OEI/OIF veterans. States seek resources such as screening and assessment tools and training, particularly on PTSD, TBI, and the military culture.

New York, Connecticut, and New Mexico believe that providers are capable of addressing the substance use treatment needs of this population, but are concerned that providers need to be trained on how to recognize and/or address associated issues like PTSD and TBI. Specifically, States have been looking, unsuccessfully, for screening and assessment tools for PTSD and TBI, and corresponding trainings to teach their providers to use such tools. In addition, the responsibility for conducting trainings for primary care physicians on how to identify PTSD and TBI and make appropriate referrals often falls on the substance use/mental health division in a State. A major initiative in nearly all of the States is the cross-training of providers (e.g., primary care providers and SUD providers) focused on how to identify and assess PTSD and TBI.

Connecticut, North Carolina, and Oregon identified trauma training, which addresses methods to treat co-occurring SUD and PTSD, as an important component of helping providers and partner agencies address the SUD needs of returning veterans and their families. All of these States currently train providers who work with veterans on the Seeking Safety model (Najavits, 2002), but they believe that something specific to veterans' trauma would be more useful.

Another common training that States are working to develop is "Military 101" training. Currently Connecticut and New York offer trainings on military culture to providers. The States that have implemented this training believe that providers will be better equipped to understand the experiences of their clients, less likely to inadvertently retraumatize clients, and better able to communicate with clients after participating in these trainings. A related training that States are providing more informally is about understanding TRICARE, the VA systems, and VA benefits.

The SSAs in Connecticut, New York, Oregon, and Utah are working across systems as part of jail diversion programs. SSA staff in each of these States has provided, or is planning to provide, outreach and trainings to law enforcement officials, the courts, emergency medical technicians, and hospital workers about the specific needs of veterans and their families. Often, domestic violence workers are included in these initiatives. However, trainings on recognizing SUDs, PTSD, and TBI for these groups have not yet been developed in most States.

No States are providing trainings to providers specifically on conducting prevention among returning veterans and their families. Both New York and North Carolina provide school-based outreach and prevention to the children of OEF/OIF veterans, and several States participate in predeployment prevention for National Guard members with their States' National Guard units and their National Guard members' families.

Common Barriers

There are many barriers to SUD treatment for returning veterans and their families. The most common barriers cited by the case study States were funding, transportation, and collaboration with and knowledge of VA.

Due to the current budget situation, many SSAs are facing level or reduced budgets. Limited funding is a major barrier to providing additional trainings to substance use providers, primary care physicians, and others. Some States have been able to leverage dollars within their region to create regional trainings through the ATTCs. Other ATTCs have used their Federal funding to create such trainings.

Materials from these trainings, and agendas from conferences held by ATTCs, are included in Appendix C.

Transportation was cited as a major barrier in every State (including even the small State of Rhode Island). This problem is exacerbated in large rural States like Wyoming, Utah, Oregon, and New Mexico. New Mexico Behavioral Health Collaborative staff noted that OEF/OIF veterans spent a great deal of their combat time in a vehicle, and many experienced traumatic events in a vehicle. For these veterans, specifically, there is a danger that they will be retraumatized or suffer a flashback while being transported for services. In addition, for many of the veterans served by the publicly funded addiction treatment system, a long commute to treatment is a major financial burden. This is particularly a problem for veterans who are eligible for or enrolled in TRICARE. TRICARE's network is limited, and in most States, veterans with TRICARE eligibility are not eligible for services in the publicly funded treatment system, and are therefore unable to receive community-based services. In Connecticut, New Mexico and Oregon, lack of nearby VA facilities (and transportation to such facilities) have been recognized as a major barrier to treatment, and veterans are eligible to receive publicly funded services, even if they have TRICARE or other health insurance benefits. These policies are financial drains on the publicly funded system, which is not reimbursed by the VA for providing services to veterans.

To alleviate this problem, five States are using or are hoping to invest in telehealth services, which will allow returning veterans to receive SUD services remotely. Connecticut currently uses a call center to provide referrals to community-based services, and New Mexico's Behavioral Health Collective has a designated telehealth unit housed within a VA facility and using VA psychiatrists. In addition to easing transportation problems, telehealth allows for anonymity for veterans who are receiving substance use services.

Transportation is a barrier, not only to getting services for veterans and their families, but also to conducting trainings to providers. Like their clients, SUD treatment and prevention providers find traveling across the State to be a major burden. To address this problem, States are increasingly turning to web-based trainings through podcasts, webinars, and webcasts. North Carolina has begun to offer training podcasts to reduce costs. New York has found that providing a combination of online workbooks and webinars has been effective in training providers on a variety of subjects, including the substance use needs of returning veterans and their families. They are hoping to develop webcasts, which will allow them to increase participation in webinars from 400 participants to an infinite number of participants, and will allow providers to access the webcasts at times that are convenient for them. Pennsylvania is also utilizing web technology to provide trainings and updates to their providers.

Other barriers cited by the case study States included the need for better collaboration between the SSA and the VA (Connecticut and Pennsylvania) and a lack of knowledge regarding resources and benefits for veterans and their families, both among veterans and among community-based SUD providers (Oregon, Utah, and Wyoming).

Key Issues

In each of these nine States, the SSA noted strong leadership from their Governor and State funding for programming that addresses the needs of returning veterans and their families, ranging from about $500,000 in Wyoming to S1.5 million in New Mexico. Each of these States initiated such projects by working with a Governor's task force and with other State agencies that serve this population. Informants noted the importance of cross-systems collaborations. Specifically, States noted that their partnerships with the VA are particularly effective in addressing the substance use service needs of returning veterans. States that work collaboratively believe that they have improved engagement rates.

Connecticut, New York, and Rhode Island emphasized their "no wrong door approach," which means that regardless of what system the veteran or his or her family presents to, they will be assessed and steered toward a menu of appropriate services, including SUD services. In this approach, the importance of coordination with and linkages to other systems and agencies to let them know what services are available is paramount. With this information, these agencies can make referrals and conduct outreach on behalf of the SSA to their clients.

Specific mention was made by Connecticut, New York, Pennsylvania, Rhode Island, and Wyoming about the importance of coordination, communication, and linkages between the SSA and the VA. After working with its VA counterparts, Connecticut found that SSA staff/providers were able to help returning veterans engage in SUD services provided by the VA, rather than only making referrals. In addition, community-based clinicians in Connecticut have successfully worked with their VA counterparts to conduct discharge planning to assist veterans' transition back into the community.

States also noted that, often, veterans are unaware of the benefits that are available to them, both within the VA system and in the community-based system. North Carolina has a web-based resource center to provide information about all services available in their States to returning veterans and their families, and Oregon is considering creating a true one-stop referral bulletin board on the internet to better educate returning veterans and their families about the mental health, SUD, TBI, and PTSD services available to them. Wyoming emphasized the importance of helping returning veterans and their families find safe, permanent housing and providing financial counseling to allow them to create stability in their lives while addressing SUDs. In addition, New Mexico, New York, and Oregon noted the importance of addressing the holistic needs of veterans and their families.

LESSONS LEARNED

During the course of the case studies, several lessons were learned. Specifically, NASADAD learned that initiatives for returning veterans are relatively new and varied; there is a large need to analyze the specific needs of OEF/OIF returning veterans and their families and to evaluate the specific initiatives for veterans. States are increasingly looking to the internet to provide and improve SUD treatment to returning veterans and their families.

Though States have treated veterans within their systems for decades, these States did not begin their current dedicated initiative to address the needs of returning veterans and their families before 2005. Pennsylvania and Rhode Island both began their initiatives in that year; Connecticut, New Mexico, Utah, and Wyoming began working on their initiatives in 2007; and New York and Oregon began their current programs in 2008. Because very limited data are available on the numbers of individuals served, types of services delivered, and client outcomes, additional evaluation of State efforts is required in the future.

In addition, there are few nationally recognized trainings, or manualized, evidence- based practices that States have been able to adapt for their own systems. As publicly funded, community-based SUD providers treat increasing numbers of returning veterans and their families, it is important to identify cost-effective, evidence-based practices to serve this population most efficiently. The only State that is conducting a rigorous evaluation of its dedicated programming is New Mexico.

Finally, as trainings are developed, it is important to consider that States are increasingly using web-based systems to provide treatment to returning veterans and trainings to providers. States believe that telehealth services are cost-effective and minimize transportation and distance barriers. In addition, SUD services provided via telehealth systems minimize stigma by increasing anonymity, which is very attractive to many returning veterans and their families.

States are also using web-based technology to conduct trainings for substance use providers. Like returning veterans and their families, it is expensive for SUD providers to travel to trainings. Additionally, they lose much-needed revenue because of their unavailability to provide services to their clients. States have been able to provide web-based trainings to providers that reduce this barrier. Currently, most States are using webinar technology, but webcast technology would allow providers to complete online trainings at times that are most convenient to them.

CONCLUSION

As more veterans and active duty military return from combat, the publicly funded substance use prevention, treatment, and recovery system and the office of the SSA will be increasingly called upon to provide services to this population and their families. In anticipation of this, Partners for Recovery (funded by SAMHSA) is working to ensure that the substance use service workforce is prepared to serve veterans that access the community-based system. As a first step in this process, NASADAD conducted a brief environmental scan of selected States to learn about specific trainings and outreach initiatives being offered by the SSA to substance use treatment and prevention providers to help them better serve returning veterans. To accomplish this, NASADAD conducted case studies of nine States that had been identified as having the largest number of initiatives for returning veterans. The data for these case studies were gleaned from interviews with SSA staff and staff from publicly funded SUD treatment facilities, during which NASADAD staff gathered data on State policies, trainings, and outreach efforts, as well as recommendations for future development of technical assistance and training materials to address the gaps in services.

Upon review of these case studies, several training needs have become apparent. Most importantly, States requested trainings for substance use services providers, as well as primary care providers, to identify and treat PTSD and TBI as well as veteran-specific trauma (military sexual trauma). States are working to identify appropriate screening and assessment tools for PTSD and TBI. Once these tools are identified, States will need to train their providers in how to use them. Many States are also responsible for training primary care physicians, law enforcement agents, and others to recognize and assess mental health disorders, SUDs, TBI, and PTSD.

The case study States emphasized the importance of treating returning veterans and their families holistically. For returning veterans and their families, this means that clinicians must have an understanding of military culture. Clinicians should also be prepared to provide or refer to a variety of community services including childcare services, financial planning services, primary care services, and safe housing. The provision of these services often requires outreach and collaboration with multiple systems.

Each of the case study States noted transportation as a major barrier to training providers and treating the SUDs of returning veterans and their families. To address this barrier in a cost-effective way, all of the States requested technical assistance to increase telehealth and webinar capabilities.

Such capabilities will also allow veterans and their families to increase their anonymity.

Finally, because best practices on addressing the SUD service needs of OEF/OIF veterans and their families are limited and difficult to acquire, States are unsure what skills providers need to successfully work with this population. Even when States are able to identify training needs, it is costly for them to develop and deliver their own trainings. This remains the largest barrier to addressing the specific needs of returning veterans and their families.

The nine States chosen for the case studies are leading the Nation in the efforts to address the unique substance use services needs of returning veterans and their families. Many other States are beginning to address this critical issue as well. Included in the nine case studies are large States and small States, representing rural and urban areas. They are geographically and politically diverse. Some have major military bases located within the State, others do not. Their diversity provides a range of rich information on State initiatives directed to serving returning veterans and their family members affected by SUDs. Further, the information gleaned from the case studies begins to identify areas where States require additional training for the workforce and related disciplines, including primary care and law enforcement, to adequately serve veterans and their families.

APPENDIX A: ADMISSIONS DATA FROM THE TREATMENT EPISODE DATA SET (TEDS)

Veterans by Age Group										
	Veterans, 18-20	Veterans, 21-24	Veterans, 25-29	Veterans, 30-34	Veterans, 35-39	Veterans, 40-44	Veterans, 45-49	Veterans, 50-54	Veterans, 55 AND OVER	All Veterans, 18+
2000	624	1,761	3,889	7,008	12,542	14,561	11,577	8,354		
2001	606	1,897	3,282	6,384	10,647	13,369	10,994	8,103	7,436	62,718
2002	654	2,047	3,238	5,945	9,926	13,608	12,251	8,959	8,186	64,814
2003	629	2,080	2,982	5,272	8,461	12,607	11,456	8,097	8,410	59,994
2004	3,184	5,458	6,656	7,898	11,110	15,716	13,774	9,308	9,761	82,865
2005	3,514	6,400	7,942	8,183	11,170	15,872	15,487	10,248	11,008	89,824
2006	2,204	4,871	6,756	6,469	9,654	14,393	16,157	11,684	12,276	84,464
2007	748	2,713	4,546	4,370	6,938	10,834	13,379	10,487	11,795	65,810
Total	12,163	27,227	39,291	51,529	80,448	110,960	105,075	75,240	76,676	578,609

Veterans Admitted to the Public Substance Use Disorder Treatment System in the Case Study States (no TEDS data for Oregon, Rhode Island, and Utah)

Connecticut								
	2000	**2001**	**2002**	**2003**	**2004**	**2005**	**2006**	**2007**
Veterans, Age 18-29	215	165	175	229	261	318	245	264
Veterans, Age 30-44	1584	1295	1136	1025	935	822	761	605
Veterans, Age 45+	1333	1163	1178	1013	881	990	925	895
% of all admissions who were veterans	7.0%	5.9%	5.8%	5.5%	5.4%	5.5%	5.0%	4.7%
New Mexico								
Veterans, Age 18-29	50	32	27	37	20	25	26	47
Veterans, Age 30-44	142	191	159	134	65	96	136	133
Veterans, Age 45+	115	173	173	124	80	136	255	248
% of all admissions who were veterans	6.5%	6.0%	6.2%	6.0%	5.0%	4.8%	5.5%	5.7%
New York								
Veterans, Age 18-29	979	902	959	822	803	924	1310	1192
Veterans, Age 30-44	6888	6420	6000	5309	4307	4196	5201	4559
Veterans, Age 45+	5279	5503	5651	5431	5141	5338	7870	7605
% of all admissions who were veterans	6.6%	6.4%	6.0%	5.5%	5.3%	4.7%	4.7%	4.5%
North Carolina								
Veterans, Age 18-29	150	159	123	72	92	81	66	81
Veterans, Age 30-44	863	802	687	581	498	409	297	333
Veterans, Age 45+	709	702	656	626	609	576	415	479
% of all admissions who were veterans	7.0%	6.3%	5.8%	5.4%	5.2%	4.8%	4.6%	4.4%
Pennsylvania								
Veterans, Age 18-29	296	259	207	193	318	228	259	267
Veterans, Age 30-44	1705	1431	1156	975	1128	794	728	711
Veterans, Age 45+	1347	1156	1029	988	1178	1047	976	858
% of all admissions who were veterans	5.3%	4.7%	3.9%	3.3%	3.0%	2.7%	2.7%	2.7%
Wyoming								
Veterans, Age 18-29	51	63	48	80	60	64	36	37
Veterans, Age 30-44	138	162	163	1745	1575	1593	1311	1179
Veterans, Age 45+	181	171	180	176	156	182	104	93
% of all admissions who were veterans	8.8%	6.9%	7.7%	6.8%	6.2%	6.3%	4.5%	4.6%

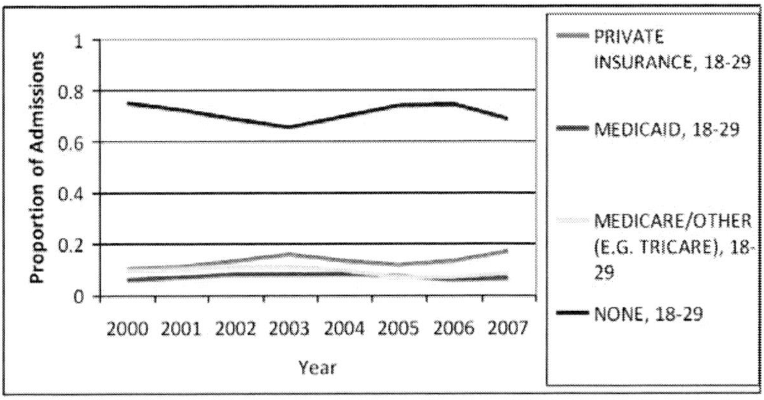

Medical Insurance Coverage of Young Veterans at SA Treatment Admission, 2000-2007.

APPENDIX B. DISCUSSION GUIDE

Addressing the Substance Use Disorder (SUD) Service Needs of Returning Veterans and Their Families

The Training Needs of State Substance Abuse Agencies (Single State Agencies, or SSAs) and Their Providers

NASADAD staff will interview key stakeholders from nine States to understand the State's current initiatives for OEF/OIF Veterans. In each of the nine States, NASADAD staff will interview: the SSA; the NTN; the person responsible for trainings or CEUs; the person in charge of services for veterans in the SSA's office (if such a person exists in any of the chosen States); and possibly a provider who would be identified by the SSA's office who has participated in the States' initiatives and serves returning veterans and/or their families. Topics discussed will include:

- Policy initiatives;
- Initiatives to assist providers;
- Trainings for providers;
- Outreach assistance;
- Other initiatives;
- Funding streams; and
- Data collection.

Interviews will be structured around the interview guide and will be conducted over the phone and will be targeted to last 30 minutes, with possible follow-up and clarifying questions via email. The States chosen will be the nine States (RI, NM, CT, NC, WY, UT, PA, OR and NY) that reported having undertaken the greatest number of initiatives for this population in NASADAD's July/August 2008 brief inquiry on returning veterans and their families.

1. We would like to talk to you about **policy initiatives** in your States that serve the substance use treatment and prevention needs of OEF/OIF Veterans and their families. In response to our inquiry in July/August 2008, we learned that your State has several such initiatives including _________.
   1a. Please describe the initiative.
   1b. Please describe the goals of the initiative.
   1c. Please describe your agency's role in each initiative.
   1d. How were the initiatives funded? Which agencies contributed? Was it funded with new or redistributed funds?
   1e. What were the practical implications of these policy initiatives? For example, did communication with the National Guard lead to the SSA providing materials or trainings to Guardmembers and their families?
   1f. What barriers did you encounter while trying to implement these initiatives? How were they overcome?
   1.g. Beyond the initiatives that I just mentioned, has your State implemented any other policy initiatives to better serve the substance use treatment needs of OEF/OIF Veterans? The family members of OEF/OIF Veterans?
2. We learned from our 2008 inquiry that your State has implemented several **initiatives to help providers** in your States respond to the substance use treatment and prevention needs of OEF/OIF Veterans and their families. You wrote that your State has ________.
   2a. Please describe your role in each initiative.
   2b. Was this initiative funded by the SSA, or another agency? Which other agency? Was it funded with new or redistributed funds?
   2c. What barriers did you encounter while trying to implement these initiatives? How were they overcome?
   2d. Did you work with the VA or DOD?
   2e. Were particular OEF/OIF populations targeted (branches, etc.)?

2f. How is the effectiveness of these initiatives evaluated?

2g. Beyond the initiatives that I just mentioned, has your State implemented any other initiatives to help treatment providers better serve the substance use treatment needs of OEF/OIF Veterans? Prevention providers? Family members of OEF/OIF Veterans?

3. Some States have assisted their providers by conducting **trainings for providers** to specifically help them to better serve the unique substance use treatment and prevention needs of OEF/OIF Veterans and their families. In response to our inquiry in July/August 2008, your State responded that it (had/had not) done this.

3a. Please describe any SSA-sponsored trainings for substance use disorder ***treatment*** providers to treat OEF/OIF Veterans? What topics were addressed in each training?

3b. Who was trained (# of people and their roles)? Who was the trainer and what were their capabilities? Can you please email us the training manual and agenda?

3c. Please describe your role in each training.

3d. Please describe the goals of the trainings.

3e. Were the trainings funded with new or redistributed funds?

3f. Did participants fill out evaluations of these trainings? Was the effectiveness of the training measured in any other ways?

3g. What barriers were encountered? How were they overcome?

3h. Please describe any SSA-sponsored trainings for substance use disorder ***prevention*** providers to treat OEF/OIF Veterans.

3i. Please describe any SSA-sponsored trainings for substance use disorder treatment or prevention providers to treat the ***family members*** of OEF/OIF Veterans.

3j. What other entities have provided trainings on this topic to providers in your State? Examples might include the National Guard, the ATTCs and others.

3k. What are the unmet training needs of providers in your State with regards to serving OEF/OIF Returning Veterans and their families? What barriers exist that prevent States from receiving this training?

3l. How did you determine who to train?

3m. How did you market the events (listerv, etc.)?

4. We are interested in learning about the ways that your State has **helped providers to conduct outreach** for OEF/OIF Veterans and

their families who might be in danger of developing, or have already developed a substance use disorder. In response to our inquiry in July/August 2008, we learned that your State has assisted providers to conduct outreach in these ways: ________.

4a. Did the State fund the outreach, and/or play a more active role?
4b. If the State played a more active role, please describe the role of the State.
4c. If the State funded the outreach, was the outreach funded with new or redistributed funds?
4d. Is outreach targeted to veterans who do not have access to services (e.g., not eligible for VA or DOD services)? Please describe.
4e. If known, please describe the outreach methods used by providers in your State.
4f. How is the effectiveness of these outreach efforts evaluated?
4g. What barriers were encountered? How were they overcome?
4h. Beyond the initiatives that I just mentioned, has your State assisted providers to conduct outreach on available substance use disorder treatment services to OEF/OIF Veterans? Substance use disorder *prevention* services?
4i. Please describe any additional assistance that your State has provided to help providers conduct outreach to the families of OEF/OIF Veterans.

5. In response to our inquiry in July/August 2008, we learned that your State has several **other initiatives** to improve substance use disorder treatment and prevention services, and access to such services for OEF/OIF Returning Veterans and their families, including ________.

5a. Has your State participated in any other initiatives to improve services and access to services for OEF/OIF Returning Veterans? If so, please describe them.
5b. Were particular veterans targeted?
5c. Please describe your role in each initiative (including the ones noted in the 2008 survey).
What were the goals of the initiatives?
5d. If funding was provided, were they funded with new or redistributed funds?
5e. Did you work with or receive funding from the VA or DoD?
5f. How was the effectiveness of each initiative measured?
5g. What barriers were encountered? How were they overcome?

5h. Has your State participated in any other initiatives to improve services and access to services for the *family members* of OEF/OIF Returning Veterans? If so, please describe them.

6. What data do you collect on veterans?
   6a. Do you specifically identify OEF/OIF Veterans as well as veterans from other wars?
   6b. Do you collect data on what branch of the military they are or were in?
   6c. Do you ask whether they are active or inactive?
   6d. Are there any other data elements that you collect on OEF/OIF veterans?

APPENDIX C. LIST OF RESOURCES BY STATE

Connecticut

Findings on the Aftereffects of Service in Operations Enduring Freedom and Iraqi Freedom and the First 18 Months Performance of the Military Support Program

PowerPoint on Veterans' Jail Diversion Program

Veterans Resource Representative Training Handbook

New Mexico

VFSS Annual Evaluation Report, 2008

New York

Action Plan for Returning Veterans and Their Families (New York State) Developed During SAMHSA's Policy Institute on Returning Veterans

Veterans Fast Facts from the New York State Office of Alcoholism and Substance Abuse Services Data Warehouse

Learning and Development Initiatives for Addiction Providers Working With Veterans – New York State Office of Alcoholism and Substance Abuse Services

Addiction Medicine Educational Series Workbook: Traumatic Brain Injury and Chemical Dependency Connection – New York State Office of Alcoholism and Substance Abuse Services

Brain Injury in the Community: Wounded Warriors in Transition (Brain Injury Association of New York State)

Institute for Professional Development in the Addictions – Veterans Roundtable at Fort

Drum Commons Presentations

Letter from the organizers

Agenda

Access to Veterans Affairs Health Care for OIF OEF Service Members – Veterans Affairs New York Harbor Healthcare System

New York Department of Veterans Affairs

Using TRICARE at the Veterans Affairs Medical Center – Veterans Affairs New York Harbor Healthcare System

What Every Clinician Should Know About Posttraumatic Stress Disorder

Buffalo City Court Veterans Project – Western New York Veterans

Homelessness and Returning Veterans – Veterans Outreach Center

Traumatic Brain Injury in the War Zone

Veterans Affairs Healthcare for Returning Combat Veterans

Why We Serve

North Carolina

Painting a Moving Train Training Workshop Agenda and PowerPoint presentation

Interview/Registration Form: Standardized Consumer Screening-Triage-Referral

Integrated Payment and Reporting System Target Population Details – FY 2008-09: Adult Mental Health and Child Mental Health Veteran and Family Target Populations

The Governor's Focus on Returning Combat Veterans and their Families: Information Brief for Substance Abuse Professionals

Added: Citizen Soldier Demonstration Project outline

What Primary Care Providers Need to Know

Treating the Invisible Wounds of War (online tutorial)

Invisible Wounds of War/Traumatic Brain Injury Training Program

Working Miracles in People's Lives: Connecting the Faith Community and Behavioral

Health Professionals to Help Service Members and Their Families

4th Annual RAH Symposium: Operation Reentry: Rehabilitation Strategies Facing Military Personnel, Veterans, and Their Dependents

The Governor's Summit on Providing Mental Health and Substance Abuse Services to Returning Combat Veterans and their Families: Summary Report

North Carolina Web Resources

North Carolina Area Health Education Centers Program

http://www.ncahec.net/

Area Health Education Center Course: Treating the Invisible Wounds of War

http://www.aheconnect.com/citizensoldier/cdetail.asp?courseid=citizensoldier

Area Health Education Center Course: ICARE: What Primary Care Providers Need to Know About Mental Health Issues Facing Returning Service Members and Their Families

http://www.aheconnect.com/ahec/cdetail.asp?courseid=icare7

North Carolina CareLINK https://www.nccarelink.gov/ Painting a Moving Train

http://bluenc.com/painting-moving-train

Governor's Institute on Alcohol and Substance Abuse

http://www.governorsinstitute.org/

Citizen-Soldier Support Program (CSSP)

http://www.aheconnect.com/citizensoldier/

Carolinas Rehabilitation - TRICARE Network Provider as a Direct Result of Citizen Soldier Support Program Traumatic Brain Injury Training

http://www.carolinasrehabilitation.org/body.cfm?id=27&action=detail&ref=37

Citizen Soldier Support Program Podcast, Part 1. 2. 3
http://www.arealahec.org/index.php?option=com_content&task=category &sectioni d=4&id=42&Itemid=100

Oregon

Governor's Task Force on Veterans' Services: Final Report (December 2008)

VHA- Oregon Medical Services PowerPoint

Portland VAMC PowerPoint

Table of Geographic Distribution of FY07 VA Expenditures in Oregon Housing, Homelessness, and Community Services PowerPoint Central City Concern PowerPoint

Worksource Oregon-Oregon Employment Department Veterans' Programs

Hire Oregon Veterans Project (HOV)

Working With Trauma Survivors PowerPoint

Oregon Department of Human Services 2009-11 Policy Option Package: Addiction Services for Uninsured Workers and Returning Veterans

Oregon Web Resource

Oregon National Guard Reintegration Team
http://www.orng-vet.org/

Pennsylvania

Serving Those Who Serve: Veterans and Their Families Brochure – Pennsylvania Regional Drug and Alcohol Training Institute (RTI)

Trauma, Terrorism, and Substance Abuse NeATTC Newsletter

Traumatic Brain Injury – Institute for Research, Education, and Training in Addictions (IRETA)

Veterans and Homelessness Training Session Information – IRETA

Treatment for Veterans with PTSD, Secondary Stress and Addiction Issues – IRETA

Pennsylvania Web Resources

PACARES
http://www.pacares.org/

Pennsylvania Department of Military and Veterans Affairs
http://www.milvet.state.pa.us/DMVA/index.htm

IRETA
http://www.ireta.org/

Rhode Island

The Rhode Island Blueprint: Addressing the Needs of Returning Soldiers and Their Families

Rhode Island Web Resource

Virtual Bulletin Board for Information for Female Veterans in Rhode Island http://www.dhs.ri.gov/Veterans/Resources/tabid/783/Default.aspx

Utah

Returning Veterans and their Families Strategic Planning Conference and Policy Academy – State of Utah Team Application

Utah Web Resource

http://www.utvethelp.com/

Wyoming

The Wyoming Department of Health Plan to the Select Committee on Mental Health and Substance Abuse: Executive Report on Veteran's Mental Health Needs

Wounded Warrior Wellness Workshop Agenda

Wyoming Web Resource

Wyoming Family Readiness Program
https://www.wy.ngb.army.mil//

Other State Resources

New Hampshire

"Coming Together: Coming Together to Better Serve Our Veterans" Agenda Article From the *Union Leader* About "Coming Together" Training

Ohio

Ohiocares Webshot/Brochure

South Dakota

South Dakota National Guard Joint Substance Abuse Prevention Program Brochure

Virginia

Virginia Is for Heroes Conference Report and PowerPoint presentations Conference Report

What Can We Learn From Col Jenny Holbert's Story

Outreach Initiatives

DoD, VA, State and Community Partnership in Service to OEF/OIF Service Members, Veterans and Their Families

Wisconsin

Returning Veterans: Combat Stress and Substance Abuse in the Wake of War

Resources List

Additional Web Resources

Brown University's Center for Alcohol and Addiction Studies

Understanding the Language of Warriors: Substance Abuse Treatment for Iraq and Afghanistan Veterans

http://www.browndlp.org/dlpannouncement.php?course=94

Great Lakes ATTC

Finding Balance After a War Zone Brochure

http://www.attcnetwork.org/learn/topics/veterans/docs/FindingBalanceBrochure.Pdf

Finding Balance After a War Zone Quick Guide for Veterans and Service Members

http://www.attcnetwork.org/learn/topics/veterans/docs/FindingBalancePocket.pdf

Finding Balance After a War Zone - Clinicians Guide (Draft)

http://www.attcnetwork.org/learn/topics/veterans/docs/FindingBalance.pdf.

MidAmerica ATTC

Pocket Resource for Policy Makers

http://www.attcnetwork.org/learn/topics/veterans/docs/PocketResouce.pdf

National Center for PTSD (www.ptsd.va.gov/index.asp)

Returning from the War Zone: A Guide for Families of Military Members

http://www.ptsd.va.gov/public/reintegration/guide-pdf/FamilyGuide.pdf

Returning from the War Zone: A Guide for Military Personnel

http://www.ptsd.va.gov/public/reintegration/guide-pdf/SMGuide.pdf

Iraq War Clinician Guide: Substance Abuse in the Deployment Environment

http://www.ptsd.va.gov/professional/manuals/manual-pdf/iwcg/iraq_clinician_guide_v2.pdf

Northeast ATTC

Resource Links, Vol. 6, Issue 1, Fall 2007: Issues Facing Returning Veterans

http://www.attcnetwork.org/learn/topics/veterans/docs/VetsNwsltr2007.pdf

Resource Links, Vol. 3, Issue 1, Summer 2004: Substance Use Disorders and the Veterans Population

http://www.attcnetwork.org/learn/topics/veterans/docs/vetnwsltr2004.pdf

Resource Links, Vol. 1, Issue 1, April 2002: Trauma, Terrorism and Substance Abuse http://www.ireta.org/attc/resources/newsletters/rl_1-1_trauma.pdf

Northwest Frontier ATTC
Addiction Messenger: Returning Veterans Journey, Part 1, Awareness
http://www.attcnetwork.org/learn/topics/veterans/docs/Vol%2011Issue7.pdf

Addiction Messenger: Returning Veterans Journey, Part 2, Trauma and Substance Abuse
http://www.attcnetwork.org/learn/topics/veterans/docs/Vol%2011Issue8.pdf

Addiction Messenger: Returning Veterans Journey, Part 3, Families
http://www.attcnetwork.org/learn/topics/veterans/docs/Vol11Issue9.pdf

SAMHSA
Resources for Returning Veterans and Their Families
http://www.samhsa.gov/Vets/

References

Eggleston, A. M., Straits-Tröster, K. & Kudler, H. (2009). Substance use treatment needs among recent veterans. *North Carolina Medical Journal*, *70*, 54–48.

Hoge, C. W., Castro, C. A., Messer, S. C., McGurk, D., Cotting, D. I. & Koffman, R. L. (2004). Combat duty in Iraq and Afghanistan, mental health problems, and barriers to care. *New England Journal of Medicine*, *351*, 13–22.

Jacobson, I. G., Ryan, M. A. K., Hooper, T. I., Smith, T. C., Amoroso, P. J., Boyko, E. J. et al. (2008). Alcohol use and alcohol-related problems before and after military combat deployment. *JAMA*, *300*, 663–675.

Najavits, L. (2002). *Seeking safety: A treatment manual for PTSD and substance abuse*. New York: Guilford Press.

Seal, K., Metzler, T. J., Gima, K. S., Bertenthal, D., Maguen, S. & Marmar, C. R. (2009). Trends and risk factors for mental health diagnoses among Iraq and Afghanistan veterans using Department of Veterans Affairs health care, 2002–2008. *American Journal of Public Health*, *99*, 1651–1658.

Tanielian, T., Jaycox, L. H., Schell, T. L., Marshall, G. N., Burnam, M. A., Eibner, C. et al. (2008). *Invisible wounds of war: Summary and recommendations for addressing psychological and cognitive injuries.* Retrieved April 18, 2009, from http://www.rand.org/pubs/monographs/2008/RAND_MG720.1.pdf.

End Note

[1] These two operations are part of what is referred to as "Overseas Contingency Operation" by the current administration.

In: Understanding Military Personnel … ISBN: 978-1-62808-636-2
Editor: Aaron D. Goodman

Chapter 2

Understanding the Military: The Institution, the Culture, and the People. Information for Behavioral Healthcare Specialists Working with Veterans and Service Members*

Angela Halvorson

Introduction

The U.S. Armed Forces are highly trained and ready to respond at a moment's notice to natural or human-made disasters anywhere in the country or the world. Yet many Americans' knowledge about the military is limited to what they have acquired from movies, books, and news reports. Few outside the military understand the culture, the values, or the people who make up the most powerful military force on earth.

What do people see in the U.S. Armed Forces that makes them dedicate their lives, and their families' lives, to military service? What is the U.S. military and who are the people who fill its ranks? How have the wars in Iraq

---

* This report was released by The Substance Abuse and Mental Health Services Administration's Center for Substance Abuse Treatment, under the Partners for Recovery Initiative, 2010.

and Afghanistan affected today's Armed Forces? What does this mean for the helping professionals who would serve them after they return from deployment?

This paper is designed to answer some of these questions by providing an overview of the military as an institution, the service members and their families who are the backbone of the institution, and how current military conflicts have affected service members, their families, and the future of military service.

The information contained herein is not an exhaustive overview of military culture but provides civilians, specifically behavioral healthcare specialists working with military personnel, with a basic understanding of the unique life and culture that is the military.

U.S. Armed Forces: The Institution

Like any large organization with a well-established history, the U.S. Armed Forces has its own culture, language, and ways of conducting business. For civilians with little or no personal exposure to the military culture, the Armed Forces may seem overwhelming, incomprehensible, esoteric, or even anachronistic. However, to understand, work with, and help those who serve in the Armed Forces, it is necessary to have a general understanding of the institution.

The Structure

The U.S. military is civilian controlled, and the ultimate authority is the President of the United States, who serves as the Armed Forces' Commander in Chief, in a civilian rather than a military capacity. This power is vested in him or her through Article II of the U.S. Constitution; Article I of the Constitution, however, gives the U.S. Congress the power to declare war. This is a purposeful separation of powers instituted by the Founding Fathers that underscored a fear of large standing armies and their potential to impede a free and democratic society.

The U.S. military is an agency of the U.S. Government, whose role it is to implement the policies set by Congress and the Commander in Chief.

The Secretary of Defense (SecDef), a cabinet-level position, "is the principal defense policy advisor to the President and is responsible for the formulation of general defense policy and policy related to all matters of direct and primary concern to the DoD [Department of Defense] and for the execution of approved policy. Under the direction of the President, the Secretary exercises authority, direction, and control over the Department of Defense."[1] The DoD is the primary tenant agency inside the Pentagon and "is responsible for providing the military forces needed to deter war and protect the security of the United States."[2] The SecDef serves as second in command of the Armed Forces under the President. Next in the chain of command are the combatant commanders, of which there are 10 around the globe, each responsible for either a geographic area or specialized mission. The Chairman of the Joint Chiefs of Staff and the Service Chiefs of Staff are responsible for the readiness of the five branches of the Armed Forces and serve as the President's military advisors but do not serve in any military chain of command.

Budget

The United States has the largest defense budget in the world. In 2010, more than $550 billion was appropriated for the Department of Defense, more than a 75 percent increase over 2001 appropriations. The large increase in defense appropriations is due primarily to the cost of manning, training, and equipping two fighting forces—one in Iraq and one in Afghanistan. An additional $130 billion was appropriated for Overseas Contingency Operations. An average of an additional $200 billion was appropriated for other defense-related spending that includes funding for the Department of Veterans Affairs, Homeland Security, and the State Department.[3]

Branches of Service

There are five branches of the military—the Army, Navy, Marine Corps, Air Force, and Coast Guard—under three primary military departments: the Department of the Army, the Department of the Navy, and the Department of the Air Force. The Marine Corps is permanently within the Department of the Navy, while the Coast Guard falls under the authority of the Department of the Navy in wartime and under the Department of Homeland Security in times of peace. However, the Coast Guard is always considered one of the five branches of military service.

Components

Within the five services are two distinct components: the reserve component and the active component.

The Active Component

The active component is composed of full-time service members. These are the individuals who wear the uniform every day and are stationed all over the world, in both combat and noncombat situations. Active component service members and their families live on or near military posts or bases and are essentially transient, expecting to move every three to five years, a circumstance virtually unheard of in the civilian workforce. Duty locations are determined by the needs of the Armed Forces and the military qualifications of the service member. When they are not in combat, active component service members spend their days training for combat. Training takes place at their home station or at any number of training locations around the world. It is not unusual for an active component member to spend only one or two weeks at home out of every six to eight weeks. Training cycles are determined by their unit's deployment cycle and deployment schedule.

At most duty stations, active component service members and their families exist within a self-contained community. Military bases have their own grocery stores (commissary), shopping centers (base exchange [BX] or post exchange [PX]), food courts and other restaurants, dry cleaners, barber shops, hair salons, daycare centers, schools, and other daily amenities. For some military members it is possible to live life on a base or post and never interact with the "outside world." Active military families generally stick together, drawn to one another by shared experiences and lifestyles.

The Reserves

The term "reserve component" collectively refers to two organizations—the Reserves and the National Guard. The Reserves is a Federal reserve force that augments the active component as personnel requirements dictate. Each of the five services has a reserve force. As of September 2009, there were approximately 1.2 million individuals serving in the reserve component in all five services.

Members of the Reserves serve in a part-time capacity—generally one weekend a month and two weeks a year—unless mobilized to serve in a full-time capacity. However, within all five reserve services, there is a force of full-time support personnel who manage and maintain daily operations.

The Reserve force is controlled by the President and can be mobilized to meet the Federal needs of the nation. According to Federal law, the purpose of the Reserves is "to provide trained units and qualified persons available for active duty in the armed forces, in time of war or national emergency, and at such other times as the national security may require, to fill the needs of the armed forces whenever more units and persons are needed than are in the regular components."[4]

Reserve members generally train with units in their own communities, selecting units based on their proximity to where they live. However, based on job availability, it is not unheard of for Reservists to travel several hours to their training locations. Unlike the active component, Reservists are not expected to move their families every three to five years and can remain in one unit as long as there is opportunity for advancement.

National Guard

Similar to the Reserves, National Guard members serve in a part-time capacity—one weekend a month and two weeks a year for training. As of 2009, approximately 500,000 individuals served in the National Guard, in either the Army National Guard or the Air National Guard. Each State, territory, and the District of Columbia has its own National Guard, as provided in the U.S. Constitution. A full-time force in each State provides daily management support for National Guard units.

Guard units exist in communities across the country and are integral to community life. National Guard armories are used for community events; Guard members are included in community activities such as parades and sporting events. Local Guard units are composed of people who live and work in the community, and many communities take great pride in and ownership of their service members. This has been especially true during the wars in Iraq and Afghanistan, when large ceremonies have seen deploying service members off and welcomed them home. Because of these close ties, the communities have also been greatly affected by the deaths of service members from their communities. It is not uncommon for members to remain with the same Guard unit for most of their careers. People select units that are close to where they live and work, though, like Reservists, it may be necessary for an individual to travel some distance to a unit where there is a position that fits his or her job specialty or rank.

Unlike the Reserves, the National Guard has two missions—a Federal mission and a State mission. The Guard's primary mission is to support the States in times of natural and human-made disasters. Guard units in each state can be mobilized by the Governor to provide support within the state or, under certain conditions, across state lines. This occurs when the Governor declares a state of emergency following civil unrest or natural disaster. California activated Guard members to help fight forest fires during the spring and summer of 2009. Illinois activated Guard members in 1993, 1994, and 1995 to support local law enforcement following the riots that took place in Chicago following the Chicago Bulls' NBA Championship wins. In 2004 thousands of National Guard troops from all over the country were activated and deployed throughout the Gulf Coast region to help in the aftermath of Hurricane Katrina. The Guard responds to all types of emergencies, including snowstorms, tornados, fires, and floods, and trains regularly to support local officials in times of flu epidemics, and chemical, nuclear, or biological attacks or accidents.

While the U.S. Constitution places control of the National Guard firmly in the hands of the Governors of each state, there are legal provisions that allow the President to mobilize National Guard units for Federal service. The National Guard can be mobilized in whole or in part to support the nation in times of emergency, in response to national disasters, or in times of war. This activation can occur on American soil or overseas, though the Posse Comitatus Act of 1878 forbids the use of U.S. Armed Forces for law enforcement purposes on U.S. soil, except for the purpose of putting down rebellions or enforcing constitutional rights if state authorities fail to do so. In this instance, the President can invoke the Insurrection Act of 1807 and go above a Governor's head to activate troops. This has been done only a few times in the last several decades, including the school desegregation in 1957 following the *Brown* v. *Board of Education* Supreme Court decision, and again in 1992 during the riots in Los Angeles following the acquittal of police officers charged with beating Rodney King. In addition to their activations in support of combat operations in Iraq and Afghanistan, Guard units have taken on what were formerly active component missions in Kosovo, Bosnia, and other theaters. These are generally one-year deployments that, while not as dangerous in most cases as deployment to Iraq or Afghanistan, still require a Guard member to put his or her life on hold and deploy overseas for an extended period of time.

While it is important for civilians in the behavioral health community working with National Guard members to have an understanding of the combat experiences affecting the mental health or substance use of current and former Guard members, it is also critical to gain an understanding of any time they may have spent activated in support of natural or human-made disasters as part of their State missions. Domestic operations may be equally traumatic and psychologically damaging for service members.

The Reserves and National Guard in OIF and OEF

The National Guard and Reserves have played a role in every major U.S. armed conflict since the Revolutionary War. However, since the inception of U.S. involvement in Operation Enduring Freedom (OEF) (Afghanistan) in 2001 and Operation Iraqi Freedom (OIF) in 2003, the National Guard and Reserves have been deployed at a rate and in numbers not seen since World War II. Between 2001 and 2007, more than 250,000 Guard members and more than 200,000 Reservists were deployed to Iraq or Afghanistan, while 1.2 million active service members served in the two combat theaters. At one point, January 2, 2008, the National Guard made up 7 percent of the total force in Iraq, while the Reserves comprised 4 percent of American forces in Iraq. At the same point, the National Guard and Reserves made up 15 percent and 6 percent, respectively, of the total force in Afghanistan. [5]

Additionally, the role of the Army Reserve and Army National Guard has changed in OIF and OEF. Historically the Reserve forces have served in a strategic reserve capacity, defined as a "force in waiting, which does not expect to deploy unless and until there is a conflict."[6] However, because the operational and personnel requirements of OIF and OEF have dramatically increased the demand for troops and equipment in the two combat theaters, the U.S. Army[7] has transitioned its strategic reserve forces to operational forces. As an operational force, the Army Reserve and Army National Guard are now fully integrated into the deployment cycle.

This change from a strategic reserve to an operational force has multiple implications for reserve component soldiers. Whereas many enlisted in the Guard and Reserve to serve their country but not to serve in a full-time capacity, the increase in the deployment tempo poses significant challenges for service members and families as they attempt to deal with the longterm separation. Employers of Guard and Reserve members are also forced to overcome a year or more without an employee. While Federal law prohibits termination of a serving member of the Armed Forces and provides other employment protections for Guard and Reserve members, multiple deployments places great strain on employers of service members. Additionally, multiple deployments increase the likelihood that service members will develop mental health issues, use alcohol or other drugs, engage in increased high-risk activities, and report chronic physical pain and other health challenges. The fact that reserve component service members and their families live in the civilian community, separate from daily contact with the military culture, structure, and support, adds a degree of isolation that can exacerbate both service members' and families' psychological challenges.

Military Ranks and Chain of Command

Military rank is about leadership and responsibility. As an individual is promoted through the military ranks, he or she assumes additional responsibility for more personnel, equipment, resources, and missions/operations. Military ranks are divided into three categories: enlisted, officer, and warrant officer. Enlisted rank includes the ranks of private, corporal, sergeant, seaman, petty officer, etc. (See "Insignia of the United States Armed Forces–Enlisted" in the Appendix.) Officers are lieutenants, captains, majors, colonels, general officers, etc. (See "Insignia of the United States Armed Forces–Officers" in the Appendix.) Rank is identified administratively by pay grade. Enlisted pay grades are E-1 through E-9 ("E" for enlisted). Officer pay grades are O-1 through O-10 ("O" for officer). Warrant officers are W-1 through W-5 ("W" for warrant). There are several instances in the services in which the pay grade for a position may represent two different ranks, one with greater responsibility than the other. For example, in the U.S. Army, at the pay grade of E-4, a soldier can be either a specialist or a corporal. The rank of corporal exists primarily in combat units and denotes an individual with more responsibility than that of a specialist. In the Marine Corps at the pay grade of E-8, a Marine might be either a master sergeant or a first sergeant. A first sergeant has significantly more responsibility for personnel and is usually the senior ranking enlisted soldier in a company.

Enlisted service members comprise the "workforce" of the services. They are the men and women patrolling the streets, fixing equipment, cooking meals, processing the paperwork, and performing the thousands of tasks that keep the military functioning. Enlisted service members promoted beyond the pay grade of E-4 become noncommissioned officers (NCOs). NCOs are in charge or in control (as opposed to in command) of their units and have significant responsibility for the health and well-being of the people in a unit. It is the NCO's responsibility to ensure that service members are being fed, equipped, and trained, that they are getting enough sleep, and that they are ready to perform their mission.

Officers are commissioned by and ultimately derive their authority from the President and are confirmed by the U.S. Senate. Officers command units and are the ultimate authority and responsible party in any military unit. While they leave maintenance of troops to their NCOs, they are responsible for planning, directing, coordinating, and controlling their troops in the accomplishment of an assigned mission or operation.

Warrant officers are also considered commissioned officers and hold warrants from their service authority. Warrant officers are generally considered technical experts in a specific area. They do not hold any command authority, nor are they responsible for personnel. They are experts in maintenance, computers, aircraft, personnel functions, and other areas. The Air Force is the only service that does not have the rank of warrant officer. The Army and the Marine Corps have the rank of warrant officer one through five, while in the Navy and the Coast Guard, warrant ranks are one through four.

The Chain of Command

Each military unit from the largest (combatant commands) to the smallest (teams composed of four to five service members) has a very clear chain of command. The chain of command is based solely on the rank of the individual and there is one assigned officer in charge (the commander) and/or one enlisted or NCO at each level who bear all responsibility for the unit. As an individual meets certain benchmarks, including time in service, time at the current rank, and military education requirements, he or she is promoted up the chain of command. With each promotion up through the ranks comes additional responsibilities and greater pay. Additional responsibilities usually include oversight of a greater number of lower-ranking service members and more equipment. Regardless of rank and the number of individuals for whom a higher-ranking service member is responsible, it is the job of the man or woman in charge to ensure that his or her service members are adequately trained in their jobs, have the necessary equipment to do their jobs, are getting the necessary sleep and food to remain at peak performance, and are following the rules and regulations that dictate military performance on and off the job. If the service members are not getting what they need to perform their jobs properly, it is the commander and/or the senior ranking enlisted member or NCO who must ensure that these requirements are met.

In the civilian sector, seldom will someone under the age of 25 be placed in charge of large numbers of personnel and equipment. However, it is commonplace for newly minted second lieutenants, fresh out of college Reserve Officer Training Corps (ROTC) or other commissioning sources, to be placed in charge of 50 or more service members and thousands—or in some cases millions—of dollars' worth of equipment. They are responsible for the lives and safety of those who work for them. In a garrison (noncombat) environment, this poses little stress and minimal risk of the loss of life or property. But in a combat environment, the stress level increases exponentially and these young officers quickly lose their greenness as they are hardened by combat, death, and loss.

Each unit is clearly structured and organized based on accepted doctrine that is ingrained from the instant an individual first puts on the uniform. Individuals are immediately trained to operate within the chain of command. Each service member has a specific individual he or she reports to and who is responsible for addressing that individual's concerns or problems. "Jumping the chain of command" in most situations is strictly forbidden and may result in formal or informal disciplinary action. Going above an immediate supervisor's head is acceptable only in situations in which the lower-ranking member does not believe his or her concerns are being addressed, or in cases where the problem is with the immediate supervisor. In both instances, however, the lower-ranking member is expected to have made serious attempts to resolve the issue at the lowest level. In cases in which an immediate supervisor is believed to be abusing his or her authority, sexually assaulting or harassing subordinates, or engaging in other illegal or inappropriate behavior, junior service members are expected to report the abuses immediately to the next highest individual responsible.

Orders are issued from the top of the chain of command to the lowest-ranking members of the unit. The commander may encourage dialogue, may review recommendations for different courses of action from his or her subordinates, and may weigh various inputs in making his or her final decision; but once an order is issued, the decision is considered final. The order is executed without question. Service members who hesitate in executing an order or who publicly question an order run the risk of at least being formally or informally disciplined and at worst risking the lives of their fellow service members.

The exception the military makes for not following a direct order occurs when the order is believed to be unethical, immoral, or illegal. If an immoral or illegal order is issued, service members are bound by duty and ethical responsibility not to follow that order and to report it to the appropriate authorities.

The legitimacy of the chain of command is one of the most important characteristics of the military culture. Maintaining the integrity of the chain of command is critical to the effective functioning and mission success of the military unit. It is also designed to identify clear lines of authority and responsibility and to eliminate any confusion in the decision-making process. Living and working within the constraints of the unit chain of command dictate how an individual functions within the organization as well as how the unit functions as a whole. Those service members who are unable to work within the chain of command, who have problems with authority, or are incapable of following orders from superiors do not last long in military service and often find their time in service to be miserable and fraught with disciplinary actions.

Military Values

Honor and integrity are the core values of military service. In addition, each service has its own specific values that are taught to new recruits from the beginning of their time in service.

The Army values are:

Loyalty, Duty, Respect, Selfless Service, Honor, Integrity, and Personal Courage

Navy and Marine Corps values are:

Honor, Courage, and Commitment

Air Force values are:

Integrity First, Service Before Self, and Excellence in All We Do

Coast Guard values are:

Honor, Respect, and Devotion to Duty

The values of each of the services are more than a list of terms that young recruits must learn and repeat on command; these values define how each service member lives his or her life, approaches every duty, and succeeds at every mission. The military value system guides how each decision is made and how every operation is executed. The military value system sets the U.S. military apart from its counterparts in the civilian sector and clearly distinguishes the United States from the enemies it fights.

Leave No One Behind

In line with the military value system is the mantra that every service member knows and understands without question—"Leave no one behind." No soldier, sailor, airman, or Marine will be left on the field of battle. This means that with little regard for their own safety, service members will do everything in their power to retrieve the remains of fallen comrades, in order to ensure that they are returned to their families for burial befitting an honorably serving military member.

Military Culture

The military culture is ingrained in military personnel from the start of their careers. Everyone begins life in the military, whether active or reserve component, with some type of initial training.

The majority begin by enlisting and attending their service's basic or initial entry training or, for the Coast Guard, Navy, and the Marines—boot camp. Basic training lasts anywhere from 8 to 13 weeks depending on the service. Others enter the service through officer commissioning sources, including ROTC, one of the service academies (West Point, the Naval Academy, or the Air Force Academy), Officer Candidate School (OCS) (Army), Officer Training School (OTS) (Air Force), or by direct appointment (common in the medical professions).

Regardless of how someone enters the service, service members spend their time at initial training immersed in the military lifestyle and culture. They learn about the history of their service, military customs and courtesies, proper wear of the uniform, military bearing, military values and ethics, and other information that is critical to their success in the service, including how to listen to and follow orders and how to function within the military chain of command. Initial training teaches discipline, focus, and control. Service members are expected to be disciplined in their actions and words and to maintain control of their emotions and their physical selves at all times. Along with discipline and control comes focus. Focus is important to mission success, and the services teach young recruits how to focus in challenging situations— situations where they are lacking sleep, are physically exhausted, or are under unaccustomed and extreme stress. Learning to stay focused, in control, and disciplined in all situations are skills that service members will use throughout their military careers as they are faced with uncertain and often dangerous situations.

Another important aspect of initial training is learning to fire a weapon and protect themselves and their comrades. While the Coast Guard and the Navy focus less on warrior skills than the other three services, service members are still reminded that they may at some point be called upon to fire a weapon and possibly kill someone. The Air Force, Army, and Marines focus largely on "warrior training," or training members on skills that may be necessary in combat.

These include weapons skills—use and maintenance, hand-to-hand combat skills, and combat life-saving skills. Warrior training for young recruits underscores the fact that their first mission as soldiers, Marines, or airmen is to fight and possibly wound or kill an enemy. This training is repeated throughout a service member's career, though more in some occupational specialties than in others.

However, regardless of job function, any one in uniform may be ordered to "pull security" on a convoy or perform another mission in a combat environment in which they must be prepared to respond with deadly skill, should the need arise. These are times when all of the skills that have been ingrained in service members throughout their career are brought to bear and tested.

Service members' first introduction to military service during initial training is also where they learn that there is no greater bond than the one they share with the people "to their left and their right." For many, this bond of brotherhood/sisterhood lasts throughout their military career and beyond. This bond is highly valued, nurtured, and protected. In life-or-death situations, the people who will help pull the service members through, or who will come for them if they are wounded or killed in combat, are the people who are fighting right by their side.

ARMED FORCES: THE PEOPLE

As important as it is to understand the institutional underpinnings of the Armed Forces, it is perhaps even more important to understand the people who comprise the institution. Its members, while demographically, geographically, and ethnically diverse, share a common set of values and beliefs that today underscore their voluntary service to the nation. The U.S. Armed Forces is an all-volunteer force.

The final draft took place in December 1972, just prior to the end of the Vietnam War, following a 1971 study by the Gates Commission that supported the idea that the Armed Forces could maintain troop strength with an all-volunteer force. Since that time, although recruiting numbers have fluctuated, the U.S. military has been able to maintain a standing and ready volunteer force.

Personnel Numbers and Stationing

As of February 28, 2009, there were just over 1.4 million members serving in the Armed Forces. A breakdown by service, including the number of women as of September 2008, is listed below:

Service[8]	Officers	Enlisted	Cadets/ Midshipman	Women[9] (9/30/08)	Total (2/28/09)	Total (11/30/09)
Army	88,093	456,651	44,009	73,902	549,153	556,682
Navy	51,093	276,276	4,399	50,008	331,768	330,071
Marines	20,588	180,443	0	12,290	201,031	204,292
Air Force	64,370	261,193	4,417	64,137	329,980	334,054
Force Total					1,411,932	1,425,059
Coast Guard						43,480

As of September 30, 2009, just over 1.1 million service members were stationed in the continental United States (CONUS) and its territories, and 262,793 service members were stationed in more than 150 countries on six continents. More than 164,000 service members were stationed in Iraq, and 66,400 were serving in Afghanistan. Deployment numbers for Iraq and Afghanistan include active component, Reserve, and National Guard service members.[10]

Women in the Military

Women make up about 16 percent of the Armed Forces, significantly less than their civilian workforce counterparts at 48 percent. A total of 15 percent of the active component and 17 percent of the reserve component are females. The Marine Corps has the lowest representation of women at 5 percent, and the Air Force Reserve (23 percent) and the Army Reserve (24 percent) have the highest representation.[11] The low representation of women in the military is largely due to Federal policy that restricts women from holding certain military occupational specialties (MOS). Women are barred from serving in combat units and specialty units like the Special Forces. This exclusion policy bars women from an estimated 15–20 percent of all military occupations.[12] The National Defense Authorization Acts of fiscal years 1992, 1993, and 1994 enabled women to be permanently assigned to combat aircraft and combatant ships. Since 1994, women have been allowed to work in any unit above the brigade level. They are still barred from serving in units below the brigade level whose primary mission is direct combat operations.

Despite the prohibition against women serving in combat units, the wars in Iraq and Afghanistan have drastically changed the role of women in the military. Because most units are based in outposts spread throughout Iraq and Afghanistan, many in the middle of cities or villages, there is no clear "front line," placing women in the same daily danger as their male counterparts. Additionally, women are serving in noncombat positions traditionally held by men, like gunners in convoys where they are sitting in the turrets of military vehicles behind machine guns, "pulling security." American women have also been trained to search Iraqi women at checkpoints, exposing to them to potential enemy attacks. As a result, according to DoD statistics as of April 3, 2010, 108 women have lost their lives in Iraq and 20 in Afghanistan, while 620 women have been wounded in Iraq and 55 in Afghanistan.[13]

The wars in Iraq and Afghanistan "have cultivated a new generation of women with a warrior's ethos—and combat experience—that for millennia was almost exclusively the preserve of men. This change has occurred without the disruption of discipline and unit cohesion that some feared would unfold. ..."14 As a result of the changing role of women in the Armed Forces, the military has had to make adjustments in privacy, living arrangements, and medical care in ways never considered before 2001. U.S. men and women are co-located on bases throughout both combat theaters and, despite the initial fear that order and discipline would be compromised by males and females living in such close proximity to each other, most service members have remained professional and focused on the mission.15 In some commands, married couples are even allowed to live together, something that was unheard of just 10 years ago.

Sexual Harassment/Assault

As women play an increasing role in the U.S. military, a role that places them in almost constant close proximity to male service members, the number of reported cases of sexual harassment and sexual assaults has increased. The DoD released a report in March 2010 that found that in 2008 female service members reported 2,923 cases of sexual assault and harassment, an approximate 7 percent increase over 2007. Of the number of incidents reported, 22 occurred in Afghanistan and 141 occurred in Iraq. Some experts estimate that the number of reported assaults and incidents of harassment are underreported. The DoD has a strict no tolerance policy related to sexual harassment and assaults, yet many incidents go unreported because the victim does not want to cause trouble, may fear retaliation from the perpetrator or the perpetrator's friends, is uncomfortable about reporting the incident, just wants it to go away, or believes that nothing will be done about the incident if it is reported.

Sexual assault and harassment of military members by others in the military violates the values and ethics upon which service in the military is based. The psychological and emotional effects are multiplied when the perpetrator is someone in the individual's chain of command and is someone upon whom he or she must rely for their safety and well-being. Men and women who suffer sexual trauma are more likely to develop emotional and psychological problems and in many cases suffer from post-traumatic stress disorder (PTSD).

Demographics

The DoD publishes an annual report on social representation in the U.S. Armed Forces. The report, titled *Population Representation in the Military Services, from* the Office of the Under Secretary of Defense, Personnel and Readiness, provides data on demographic, educational, and aptitude characteristics of applicants, recruits, and enlisted and officer numbers in the reserve and active components. The following statistics have all been drawn from the DoD FY 2005 report. [16]

Age

The most recent report from FY 2005 found that the active component (AC) and reserve component (RC) service members were younger than their civilian counterparts. A total of 88 percent of AC recruits were between 18 and 24, compared to the civilian workforce at 37 percent. The mean age of AC recruits is 20. The reserve component data also showed a more youthful population than the civilian sector.

Race/Ethnicity

In the enlisted force in 2005, African Americans were proportionately represented in non-prior service (NPS) accessions at 13 percent as compared to their representation of 14 percent in the civilian population 18 to 24 years old. Other minorities, classified as American Indians, Alaskan Natives, Asian Americans, Native Hawaiians, Pacific Islanders, or individuals of two or more races, were represented at 8 percent, equal to their representation in the civilian population. Hispanics continue to be underrepresented in the Armed Forces, at 14 percent of NPS accessions compared to 18 percent of the comparable civilian population.

In the AC officer corps in 2005, minorities are proportionately represented, though African Americans make up a much smaller proportion of officers at 9 percent than they do in the enlisted ranks at 20 percent. However, in comparison to college graduates in the civilian sector (8 percent), African Americans are equitably represented. American Indians and Alaskan Natives, a very small proportion of the officer corps, are also equitably represented in comparison to the comparable civilian population of college graduates 21 to 49 years old. Hispanic officers, at 5 percent, are slightly underrepresented in the officer corps compared to their civilian counterparts at 7 percent. Asian American officers are significantly underrepresented in the officer corps at 3 percent, while their civilian counterparts ages 21 to 49 in the workforce are represented at 9 percent.

The ethnic and racial makeup of the RC is similar to that of the AC for officers and enlisted.

Education Level

The military places strong emphasis on both military and civilian education. This emphasis was apparent in the fact that in 2005 nearly all (99 percent) NPS AC and RC enlisted accessions had a high school diploma or equivalent. This is significantly higher than the comparable civilian youth population at 80 percent of youth 18 to 24 years old. In the officer corps 94 percent of officer accessions and 96 percent of the officer corps held a bachelor's degree, while approximately 15 and 38 percent, respectively, held advanced degrees. Similarly, 75 percent of the RC officer accessions and 89 percent of the total RC officer corps held a bachelor's degree, while 19 and 34 percent, respectively, held advanced degrees. The officer statistics are not surprising given the military's requirement that all officers hold at least a bachelor's degree upon or soon after commissioning.

Socioeconomic Status

The DoD has not collected socioeconomic data from recruits since 1999, though recent research conducted by the DoD has used recruits' ZIP code to attempt to categorize socioeconomic status. Using ZIP code data, DoD has found that the average socioeconomic status of recruits is similar to the civilian population.[17]

Marital Status

There had been steady increase in the number of married service members from 1973 (40 percent) to 1994 (57 percent); but that number decreased over the following 10 years to a rate of 49 percent in 2003. In 2005, the number of marriages in the service increased to 52 percent. In general, DoD found that males in the services were more likely to be married than their female counterparts. Officers are more likely to be married (69 percent AC and 73 percent RC) than their enlisted counterparts, a difference resulting from the fact that officers are generally older and more financially secure than many of the enlisted service members.

The Military Family

> "Patriotism is not a short and frenzied outburst of emotion but the tranquil and steady dedication of a lifetime."
> —Adlai E. Stevenson, Jr.

An understanding of the military family is as important to the understanding of the service member as the other aspects already described. The military family is often asked to make sacrifices well beyond any expected of their civilian counterparts. For active component family members, the military is a daily part of who they are, and the family is as much a part of the military as is the actively serving military member. Active component family members are expected to move, or PCS (permanent change of station), every three to five years. While the military is attempting to lengthen the time period in which service members and their families remain at one duty location, the reality is that the needs of the services come first, and personnel change duty locations at the pleasure of the military. With each move, family members are expected to start over—a new school, new friends, a new job, a new home, a new neighborhood, and new experiences. Pets may even have to be left behind, if the next duty station is overseas or is in a location where pets are impractical or not allowed. Housing on some bases is substandard, well below what many in the civilian community would consider acceptable, though the military is working to improve post/base housing for all ranks. For some, the normal stress of a major move is exacerbated by a parent's or a spouse's deployment soon after the PCS. In some cases spouses may move their families across the country or across the world while the service member is deployed, setting up a new home alone and without the benefit of the service member's assistance. For active service military families, the only certainty is the uncertainty they live with every day.

While military life poses many challenges for family members, how the family approaches its challenges is critical to minimizing long-term effects and building resiliency in both children and spouses. Many families view the changes not as potential negatives, but as new opportunities to be undertaken with great anticipation and excitement. Overseas moves can be looked at as opportunities to broaden horizons and expand the family's knowledge of other parts of the world. These can be wonderful experiences that few young children—and even few adults— have the chance to enjoy.

Deployments

> "Army families are the most brittle part of the force .... [They] are sacrificing too much, and we can no longer ask them to just make the best of it."
>
> —Sheila Casey, wife of Gen. George Casey, Army Chief of Staff, testifying before the Senate
> Armed Services Committee, June 2009

Day-to-day military life for family members poses many challenges. However, today's military family is dealing with the additional challenges of the deployment of one or both parents. While extended absences have long been a part of military life for family members, the current operational tempo of today's military forces has resulted in longer and more frequent deployments. Some active component family members have waited for family members to return from a third, fourth, or fifth deployment in nine years.

At a 2009 meeting of the Third Family Forum of the Association of the United States Army, Col. Kris Peterson, Army psychiatrist in charge of the Military Child and Adolescent Center of Excellence at Madigan Army Medical Center, Fort Lewis, Washington, told Army spouses and support group leaders that "...years of repeated, lengthy deployments have resulted in higher rates of anxiety and depression among Army children, as well as misbehavior in school...yearly mental health visits for children under the age of 15 have increased from 800,000 in 2003 to 1.6 million in 2008. One out of three school-age children are at risk for psychological problems and about 30 percent of children have significantly increased anxiety."[18]

While recent media attention has forced the services to take a closer look at the suicide rates of service members, the studies currently being conducted by each of the services do not include suicides and mental health issues of their families. However, there has been an increase in the number of military spouses experiencing multiple deployments who have committed suicide and who are experiencing increased depression and anxiety.[19] Despite knowing that it will only increase their anxiety, military spouses find themselves drawn to the 24-hour news reports, searching for information about their loved ones. Instant communication and Internet access allow family members at home to monitor the situation overseas almost by the minute, leaving family members virtually paralyzed with worry, yet they must also deal with the daily stressors of raising children, working, paying bills, and other responsibilities.[20] There are many related secondary effects of multiple deployments that manifest in the spouses and children of service members, and the increase in mental health needs of family members has led to a severe shortage of mental health care facilities and personnel trained to address the needs of military families, both on and off post/base. Military facilities are filled to capacity with military members, leaving family members searching for desperately needed assistance.[21]

To help address these issues, there are many supports that can help family members successfully navigate the challenges of deployments. There are multiple Web sites that offer assistance and recommendations for managing the deployment-related stresses. In addition, a National Military Family Association 2005 study recommended the following to best assist active and reserve component families through deployments: [22]

1. Address return and reunion challenges throughout the deployment cycle, not just at the end of the deployment. From the minute a service member departs, family members are imagining his or her return and reunion. Not knowing what to expect at the reunion or how to handle the reintegration increases the overall stress level.
2. Direct more resources to support family volunteers. This recommendation also included a call for additional trained counselors available through family support channels.
3. Recognize that family time is important for reintegration with family members. For active component service members especially, there is little time following deployment for them to spend quality time with their families and work on reintegration and reconnection with their families after the long separation.
4. Expand program and information outreach, and help military family members feel more connected to what is going on within the unit.

While many family members actively connect with the unit command and the unit's Family Readiness Group (FRG), there are still some who remain outside the existing support structure. It is important to reach out to those who are not connected and make attempts to help them connect with the unit support system.

5. Assist family members in setting realistic expectations for themselves, their service members, and the military unit, and then meet the expectations. Many family members expect the FRG to help them with the most mundane of tasks during the deployment, something that is not the responsibility of the FRG or of other family members. Some are afraid to ask for help for fear that it reflects poorly on themselves or on their deployed family member. It is important that the spouses and families who remain at home understand that the FRG and the military unit are there to assist them in locating the resources they need to address their needs. Family members are also entitled to many benefits and programs, of which they may not be aware. The FRG and the unit can help family members identify and apply for those benefits and programs, and help them make connections with other resources that will help them meet the many challenges associated with deployment.
6. Never assume families know what they need to know, even in situations in which the majority of family members have "done this before." This minimizes the challenges faced by family members, challenges that sometimes increase with subsequent deployments. It also discounts the number of family members who are new to the unit and who may never have experienced a deployment before.

National Guard and Reserve families face several unique challenges during a deployment that their active component counterparts do not face. Reserve component family members are unaccustomed to full-time military life and are often disconnected from the support systems that the active component has access to through their base or post. Reservists' families may be geographically separated from the unit or from the location where the FRG typically meets. If the FRG leadership does not consciously reach out to those who are not physically in attendance at meetings and activities, family members remain virtually in the dark, with little information and support to assist them in managing the stresses that are unique to having a deployed family member—stresses they are unprepared for and perhaps incapable of managing. While there may be civilian friends and family who serve as support networks, this is not the same has having fellow military family members to rely on for support. Military families have a unique understanding of the challenges and can relate in ways that civilian support systems cannot.

THE EXPERIENCE OF WAR

> "War is God's way of teaching Americans geography."
> —Ambrose Bierce

War's effects are permanent and long lasting, resulting in death and destruction that can take years or decades to overcome. War also has long-term effects on the men and women who fight and on the civilian population directly and indirectly involved in them. Everyone experiences war differently, but military service members experience many commonalities.

Physical Aspects of War

The combat zone is an intense place where things can move very quickly one moment and drag painfully slowly the next. "Hurry up and wait" is not just a phrase, but is a reality of life in a war zone. Service members move quickly to prepare for a mission and find themselves waiting for minutes or hours as plans change, intelligence is gathered, and leaders adjust decisions. Adrenaline pumps as service members gear up, load their weapons, and mount their vehicles, and then, without warning, they are told to stand down. This constant feeling of having one foot on the gas and one foot on the brake is exhausting and physically demanding, especially for troops who operate on minimum levels of sleep.

Troops are under constant physical strain that is exacerbated by unfamiliar locations, extreme heat or cold, and the 60–80 pounds of gear they are responsible for transporting, either in and out of vehicles or on their backs. Just to conduct missions in the streets or through the mountains, troops are outfitted in their protective equipment, including interceptor body armor (IBA), helmet, extra ammunition, water, weapon(s), and in some cases food. Coupled with an almost constant sense of sleep deprivation, these physical demands increase stress levels and can have a significant impact on the mental and emotional functioning of troops in combat.

Mental and Emotional Aspects of War

The physical strain is not the only thing that affects the ability of troops to function in a combat zone. There is a constant tactical awareness that keeps service members on edge and hyper-vigilant at all times. On the modern battlefield there is no front line past which the battle ensues and behind which personnel are safe. In World War I and World War II, there were clear demarcation lines indicating how far forward personnel could go before they were involved in direct combat. Rear areas were safe and out of reach of enemy guns and cannons. Thousands of support personnel remained behind the front lines and conducted their mission in support of the combat troops on the front lines. On today's battlefield, there are no clear front lines and no one—from combat troops to the support personnel—is exempt from the effects of war. Military personnel live and work on bases in the middle of a territory that might one minute be peaceful and the next erupt in a hail of gunfire. All personnel in-country are at risk of harm or death from mortars that are launched over operating base walls, sniper fire, or improvised explosive device (IED) attacks on convoys. Though it may feel safe to the troops living and working there, it is not. The environment can change without warning, forcing troops to maintain a perpetual state of vigilance and tactical awareness. Constant tactical awareness requires troops to make split-second decisions that may mean the life or death of their fellow service members. Young troops—many not older than 22 or 23 and some as young as 18—are expected to instantly read a situation, make a decision, and live with the consequences. The consequences can be life or death.

Troops in combat are faced with multiple losses, grief, and guilt that many are unprepared to deal with; and few have time to adequately process before they are back out on the next mission. In combat situations, troops may be asked to make decisions that can damage their spiritual and moral fiber, decisions that in the civilian world would have clear black-or-white answers but in the fog of war show up in hundreds of shades of grey. A service member might be forced to choose between one option that may mean the death of a (possibly) innocent civilian and another that might put his or her entire unit in jeopardy. The act of killing itself, even when it is justified and necessary, can have spiritual or moral effects at levels deeper than those decisions determined by logic or military training. Daily life is filled with uncertainty, confusion, fear, and disruption that for many are beyond their limited coping or resilience skills. This reality continues for 6, 9, 12, or 18 months.

Reunion and Reintegration

The reunion and period of reintegration that follows can be perhaps the most challenging time of a deployment. Many spouses eagerly anticipating their first moments of reunion set high expectations for what will happen. They may envision romantic evenings and a rekindling of the sexual relationship with their partner, or they may envision a spouse who returns home to help around the house and take some of the burden from their shoulders. Regardless of the high expectations, there is a strong likelihood that those expectations will be dashed, adding disappointment to the already stressful situation. Many service members return home exhausted and needing space and time to themselves. They are often withdrawn and uninterested in or incapable of physical intimacy. Some spouses return home and face their own anxieties and uncertainties. Others bring the horrors of war home with them, struggling with PTSD, nightmares, and depression. Still others may have suffered injuries, may have lost limbs, or may be suffering with traumatic brain injury (TBI) that affects their moods, personalities, cognitive abilities, and physical functioning. If infidelity was an issue during the deployment, the marriage may be failing just when the support of a loving family is most needed.

If there are children, the deployed family member is attempting to reconnect with them and to determine where he or she fits in the parental unit. Returning service members struggle with the family dynamic and what role they play in the family structure. They may have been away for more than a year, and while they may have held a specific role in the family structure before the deployment, the family member who remained at home was forced to fill this role. In some cases, the waiting family member may not be ready to relinquish this role to the returning family member, and a power struggle ensues. For example, the husband may have been in charge of managing the household finances before he deployed for a year to Iraq. Out of necessity, his wife was forced to take over this household function. She learned to manage the finances, pay the bills, and even save a little extra money while her husband was gone. The husband now wants to assume his role as family financial manager but finds his wife is unwilling to relinquish this new role. In another example, when the service member deployed, his son was an infant and barely walking and talking. When he returns, he finds a toddler with a mind and a personality of his own who needs guidance, a loving hand, and boundaries. Throughout the deployment, his wife has been raising their son. When dad returns, he not only needs to figure out how to relate to the new little being in the household, but also how to parent a toddler in partnership with his wife, while she needs to learn how to co-parent with her husband for the first time. Both these examples and countless others require adjustment to the new dynamic by both parties. If the marriage was not strong to begin with or was not nurtured by communication, honesty, and fidelity during the deployment, there is a greater likelihood of increased stress, which can lead to divorce or abuse.

During fiscal year 2009, the Department of Defense reported that the overall divorce rate for all five services increased from 3.4 percent to 3.6 percent. (The civilian divorce rate for the same time period was 3.4 percent.) Enlisted airmen reported a 4.3 percent divorce rate, the highest of all five services. However, the Army reported an increase in the divorce rate of its enlisted personnel for the seventh straight year, making it the only service to report a steady increase over that length of time. The DoD study reported the Army's divorce rate increased from 3.4 percent to 3.6 percent. The Marine divorce rate remained steady at 4 percent from 2008 to 2009. Divorce affects young enlisted members more significantly than older NCOs and officers. However, the 2009 findings reported a growing number of senior NCOs with marital problems. Army researchers have continued to study the effects of deployment on marriages, focusing efforts on troops in Iraq and Afghanistan. They have found that soldiers with greater access to electronic means of communication that allow them to interact with their family members at home are more likely to have marital problems. Researchers theorize that the more a deployed member is able to interact with his or her family, the greater the chance of becoming involved in family issues and arguments that are best left to the parent at home, or that cannot be resolved with any clarity through electronic communication.[23]

The reserve components experience reintegration differently than the active component. Whereas active service members return home to their full-time jobs as soldiers, sailors, Marines, or airmen, and to families and communities that are familiar with deployment and reintegration, the reserve components return to the civilian world and to civilian families. This poses some very unique challenges for these service members and, by extension, their families. A Guard or Reserve member still has the family reintegration challenges identified previously, but these challenges are compounded by trying to find a way to fit back into the civilian world where his or her friends and family have little direct experience with the military and little understanding of what the service member has been through. Reserve component members may be excited to return to friends who are anxious to hear about their experiences, but the initial excitement quickly wears off as a sense that everything has changed permeates relationships and other personal interactions. In fact, people have changed; the friends and family members who remained behind are different a year later, and the service member has been changed by his or her own experiences—experiences that are no longer shared with those around him or her. Once the reunion excitement has worn off, there is a desire on the part of friends and family to have things return to "normal," or as they were before the deployment. They want that person back and do not understand that the experience he or she has gone through has in many cases irrevocably changed that person. Even if the service members desperately want to "get back to normal," they no longer feel "normal" and wonder if they will ever fit in with civilian friends and family again. Many have a sense of needing to reconnect with fellow service members they served with overseas but, because of the way the Guard and Reserve are structured, they may not see their fellow service members until they return to training in 30 days or more. Guard and Reserve members may also feel a loss of mission and purpose, often returning home to roles that require less skill and authority than they exercised in their deployment roles. In-country, service members were making life or death decisions. Back home, what others see as critical pale in comparison to their combat experiences and what was important overseas. This may leave them feeling isolated and disconnected. Overseas, life had a certain intensity, routine, and pace. Yet back home, out of the military culture, that structure and routine is gone—they no longer have an operational schedule that tells individuals when to eat, when to sleep, and when they will have time to shower. What's more, combat is intense, with soldiers experiencing an almost constant adrenaline rush as they prepare for each mission. When service members return home, they feel as if their world has gone from moving from 180 miles per hour, to a dead stop.

Active component members take a couple of weeks' leave and return to life in uniform and to working side by side with the men and women they served with overseas. Reserve component members take a couple of weeks' leave, if their civilian employer is not demanding their immediate return to work, and go to work side by side with people who are untouched by combat and what is happening several thousand miles away in a distant country. In addition, reserve component members may have had positions of responsibility in their units—they were decision makers and responsible for the health and well-being of others. In their civilian employment, they may have little or no responsibility, no authority, and thus no feeling of self-worth compared to how they felt in their military position.

Access to medical care may also be a challenge for Reserve and Guard members. While the active component has access to medical and behavioral healthcare services on base or on post where they are stationed, Reservists may be geographically separated from any military healthcare facility by several hours. Now faced with redeployment issues, e.g., substance use, mental health issues, marital and family difficulties, the Reserve requires service members to attend mandatory training every 30, 60, and 90 days following redeployment. Additionally, service members are assessed to monitor how they are adjusting. Family members also undergo training and are able to connect with professionals who can help them or answer questions.

Clinical Implications

Due to improvements in protective equipment and battlefield medical care, fewer troops are dying from combat-related injuries. As a result, service members, who in previous conflicts would not have survived, are returning home wounded,[24] suffering with severe physical injuries like blindness, amputations, and burns, and also with debilitating psychological and emotional wounds. Some are even faced with "poly-trauma" in which they are suffering from multiple and complex combinations of injuries. Service members are able to access services through the Veterans Administration but many, particularly National Guard and Reserve members, are accessing primary and behavioral health services in the civilian sector.

In order to effectively treat service members who walk through their doors, civilian providers need to understand the implications of military service and combat experiences. Included in the Appendix is a matrix of experiences/conditions and the clinical implications that can be used by behavioral healthcare providers to assist service members seeking services. This list is not exhaustive but is a starting place for clinicians to begin their work with veterans and service members.

Conclusion

We are seeing unprecedented numbers of service members returning from Iraq and Afghanistan in need of behavioral healthcare services. While the Veterans Administration (VA) provides high-quality services, many service members do not go to the VA for help but instead seek assistance through the civilian sector. Because of the numbers of military men and women entering the civilian sector, civilian behavioral healthcare specialists need to have a basic understanding of this population. This paper has provided an overview of the military, its culture, and its people and can be used as one resource to build the knowledge base of individuals not familiar with the military. Additional resources are available from a variety of sources, including the Department of Defense and the Veterans Administration.

APPENDIX

Challenges and Implications for Behavioral Healthcare Services

Difficulties with Access and Reimbursement

Challenges Related to Military Service

1. Difficulties with access, understanding what services are available, and reimbursement for service members and families

Implications for Behavioral Health Services

1. Provide education, outreach, case management, and expanded services to assist service members and families in accessing needed services.

Physical (Neurological, Somatic, etc.) Effects of Life in a War Zone

Challenges Related To Military Service

1. Endocrinological and neurochemical effects of war, e.g., sleep deprivation, constant tactical awareness, etc.
2. Effects of physical strain on musculoskeletal, gastrointestinal, immune functioning, somatic experience of tension, etc.
3. Implications of the war experience and its aftermath for substance use, abuse, and addiction include:
   - The widespread use of enormous amounts of caffeine
   - Increased vulnerability to opioid addiction from pain medication
   - The temptation to use alcohol and drugs as substitutes for psychotropic medications

4. Service members and veterans are often unaware that they have experienced mild traumatic brain injury (MTBI) because they were some distance from the blast; however, they may still experience concussion and post-concussion syndrome
5. MTBI and post-traumatic stress disorder (PTSD) symptoms can be hard to distinguish, making differential diagnosis difficult

Implications for Behavioral Health Services

1. Teach and practice skills in managing stress before attempting to address deeper memories or psychological issues or maintain abstinence from alcohol and other drugs.
2. Provide or encourage a holistic approach that includes physical relaxation activities such as yoga, exercise, dancing, walking, etc.
3. Identify the chemical excesses or deficiencies that service members and veterans are attempting to balance (or, in the case of caffeine and the adrenaline rush, prolong) with chemicals, and address those excesses and deficiencies. Educate about the effects of caffeine on sleep cycles. Explore alternative pain management techniques for people addicted to pain medications. Monitor the effects of and interactions among medications, and work with prescribers to find acceptable solutions.
4. Ask questions about their proximity to blasts, and help them understand the effects of blasts even on people who are several feet away.
5. Assess for both conditions and, when in doubt, treat both conditions. Treat the whole human being, and treat according to symptom clusters.

Psychological Effects of Life in a War Zone

Challenges Related to Military Service

1. Effects of multiple losses, in traumatic circumstances, with inadequate time for grieving
2. The psychological effects of killing and harming others, although within the call of duty, and guilt caused by lives they were unable to save
3. The fact that some service members' and veterans' moral and tactical decision-making processes may have been affected by sleep deprivation

and the effects of combat stress, resulting later in increased levels of confusion, guilt, and mistrust of self

4. Effects of military sexual trauma (sexual harassment and aggression), exacerbated by the insularity of the unit culture and the betrayal of trust by comrades or commanders whose fidelity was so closely linked to emotional and physical survival

Implications for Behavioral Health Services

1. Create an atmosphere that is safe and comfortable for grieving when the service member is ready.
2. Let service members or veterans decide when to bring up issues related to harming others or guilt, rather than directing them toward them (through questions, comments, etc.). Help them see their own responsibility for what happened in context and perspective, and to separate responsibility from guilt. Help them both separate grief from guilt and understand the ways in which these experiences can complicate one another. When they are ready, help them find ways of making amends that fit their own experiences and value systems.
3. Help service members and veterans understand and accept some of the normal ways in which sleep deprivation and combat stress may affect people's thoughts, decisions, and emotions. Help them see the physical (neurochemical) roots of these effects.
4. In addressing sexual trauma issues, keep in mind the intensity of the bond between service members, the profound effects of betrayal, the effects of rank differential on these experiences, and the fact that service members are often isolated within their units.

Issues Related to Military Rank and Authority

Challenges Related to Military Service

1. Promotion in rank and decision-making responsibilities at young ages (sometimes when individuals' executive functions are not fully developed)
2. Severity of disciplinary measures that veterans and service members may have encountered in military service

Implications for Behavioral Health Services

1. If service members or veterans are experiencing stress and anxiety with the effects of early responsibilities, help them see their decisions in the context of their youth and levels of experience at the time.
2. If veterans or service members are suffering from the effects of disciplinary measures, help them distinguish between appropriate discipline and abuse of authority and address those issues separately.

Other Issues That Can Impede Help Seeking and Therapeutic Processes

Challenges Related to Military Service

1. Still-widespread military (and societal) stigma toward combat/operational stress effects, including PTSD, substance use disorders, and psychiatric disorders in general, and toward the idea of receiving help or therapy
2. Military emphasis on discipline and control, and the reluctance to experience normal emotional reactions and the emotional risks involved in the healing process

Implications for Behavioral Health Services

1. Help service members, veterans, families, communities, and the public in general understand that these are normal reactions to life in the war zone, by helping them understand the physical (e.g., neurochemical, endocrinological) roots of post-deployment stress effects. Frame services in terms of training rather than therapy, helping service members and veterans learn to manage their stress systems so they can be more effective within the civilian world. Present a performance-optimization model compatible with the military culture.
2. Establish a partnership in which service members and veterans have control over the planning and decisions that occur throughout the therapeutic process. Teach skills in managing thoughts and emotions to increase their sense of control and mastery.

Issues Related to Families and Family Reintegration

Challenges Related to Military Service

1. The importance of families' well-being to service members, and the effects of worrying about family members

2. Need for marriage (partner) and family support and/or therapy during the reintegration period
3. The importance of providing prevention, intervention, and treatment for family members, and the effects of many conditions (worry, loss, absence, isolation, disruption, etc.) on families

Implications for Behavioral Health Services

1. Provide or recommend services to family members. Understand that, even if a service member or veteran is experiencing severe problems, assisting family members may be of equal or greater priority to the service member before he or she can accept help.
2. Communicate the fact that reintegration is difficult and it is normal to need support. Help veterans, service members, and families develop support networks. Provide marriage or family therapy or make appropriate and supportive referrals.
3. Provide assistance to families before, during, and after deployment, and throughout the reintegration period, or find and make appropriate referrals. Promote community support for families of reserve component service members by engaging in community education and organizing efforts.

Issues Related to Reintegration into Civilian Culture

Challenges Related to Military Service

1. Loss of the clarity and comfort provided by the military structure, chain of command, and routine
2. Alienation from civilian culture and difficulty trusting civilians, resulting in the loss of potential support structures
3. Sense and/or appearance of being "shut down," emotionally numb or "dead," and closed off from their own emotions and from communication with civilians
4. Loss of the intense sense of mission and purpose that many experienced during deployment, often exacerbated by coming home to unemployment or employment in roles that require far less skill and authority than they exercised in their deployment roles

Implications for Behavioral Health Services

1. Help veterans or service members find or build clarity and structure, and learn to manage their discomfort with greater uncertainty and lack of structure.
2. Take great care to establish, earn, and keep service members' and veterans' trust in therapeutic relationships (including relationships with staff at all levels of the organization). Help service members and veterans understand that their sense of alienation and mistrust is normal and is not caused by deficiencies in them or in their loved ones. Help them identify those people who do deserve and will not betray their trust, deepen those relationships gradually, and manage their relationships with people whom they have reason not to trust. Encourage them to make or keep connections with other service members and veterans.
3. Understand modes of "resistance" as important forms of psychological protection. Let veterans or service members progress at their own pace through the process of opening up in therapy. Help them understand the physiological factors (e.g., excesses of parasympathetic chemicals, depletion of sympathetic chemicals) that may be contributing to their feelings of being shut down, numb, or dead.
4. Respect the sense of mission and purpose that service members or veterans experienced, whether or not it fits with the counselor's or therapist's own sense of mission and purpose. Help them explore ways of building and exercising mission and purpose back home. Connect the service member or veteran with career development resources that will help them find more meaningful work.

Using Military Values to Increase Motivation within the Therapeutic Process

- *Loyalty* - Loyalty to themselves and their families can be a good motivator to enter and make progress in therapeutic processes.
- *Respect* - Many of the symptoms of untreated combat stress and substance use disorders result in behavior that is disrespectful to the service member or veteran, the family, the military, and society as a whole. Working on these conditions and reducing their symptoms can enhance respect.

- *Selfless service* - The symptoms of untreated disorders can impair people's ability to be of service. Accepting help will improve service members' and veterans' ability to be of service.
- *Honor and integrity* - The symptoms of untreated disorders can often influence people to act in dishonorable and dishonest ways. Progress in overcoming these disorders can strengthen one's honor and integrity.
- *Excellence and commitment* - People with a commitment to excellence can use that commitment to approach the work of stress management, growth, and healing.
- *Personal courage* - The process of admitting, confronting, and learning to manage the effects of combat and operational stress requires great personal courage. Any step in this direction is a sign of courage.
- *Devotion to duty* - Service members and veterans function as individuals, family members, community members, and citizens. They have a duty to operate responsively and appropriately.

MILITARY RANKS

Insignia of the United States Armed Forces — Officers

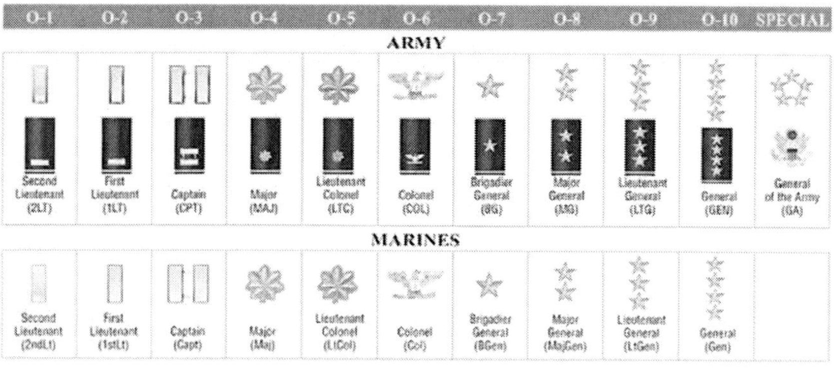
O-1
O-2
O-3
O-4
O-5
O-6
O-7
O-8
O-9
O-10
SPECIAL
ARMY
Second Lieutenant (2LT)
First Lieutenant (1LT)
Captain (CPT)
Major (MAJ)
Lieutenant Colonel (LTC)
Colonel (COL)
Brigadier General (BG)
Major General (MG)
Lieutenant General (LTG)
General (GEN)
General of the Army (GA)
MARINES
Second Lieutenant (2ndLt)
First Lieutenant (1stLt)
Captain (Capt)
Major (Maj)
Lieutenant Colonel (LtCol)
Colonel (Col)
Brigadier General (BGen)
Major General (MajGen)
Lieutenant General (LtGen)
General (Gen)

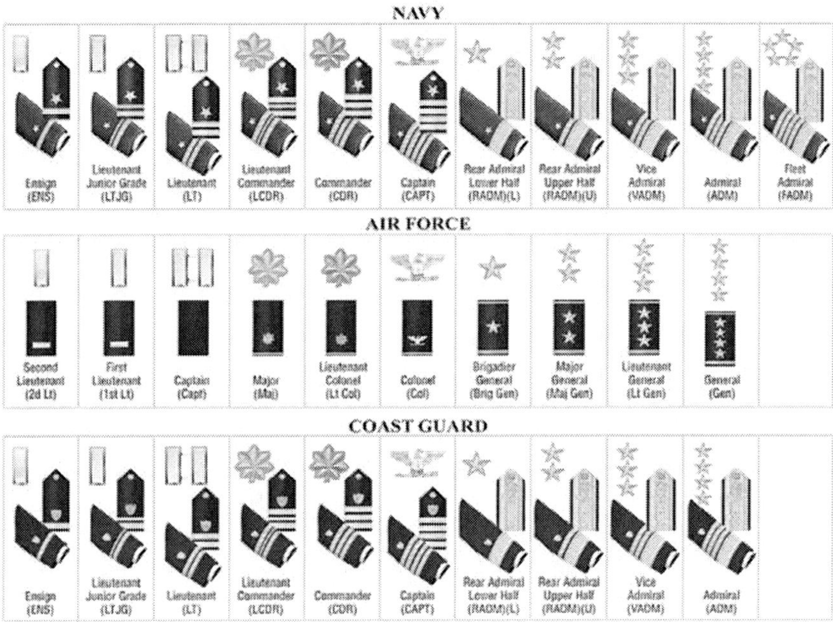

Insignia of the United States Armed Forces — Enlisted

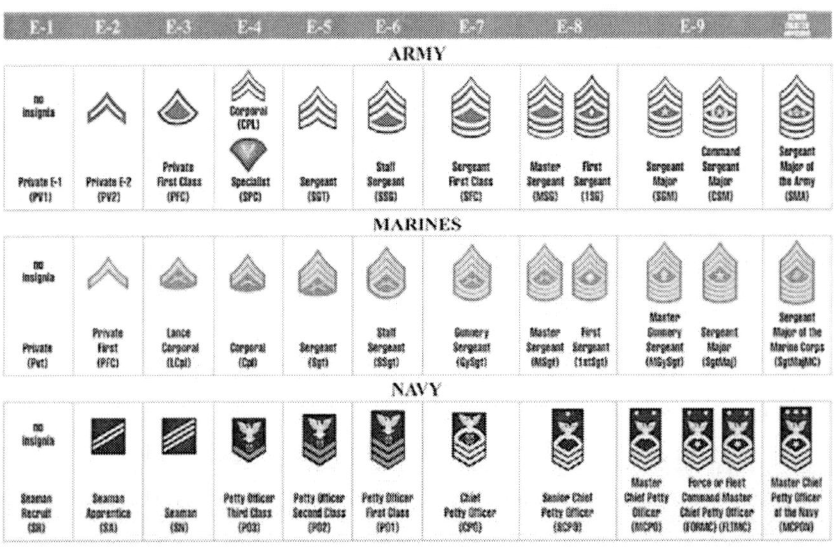

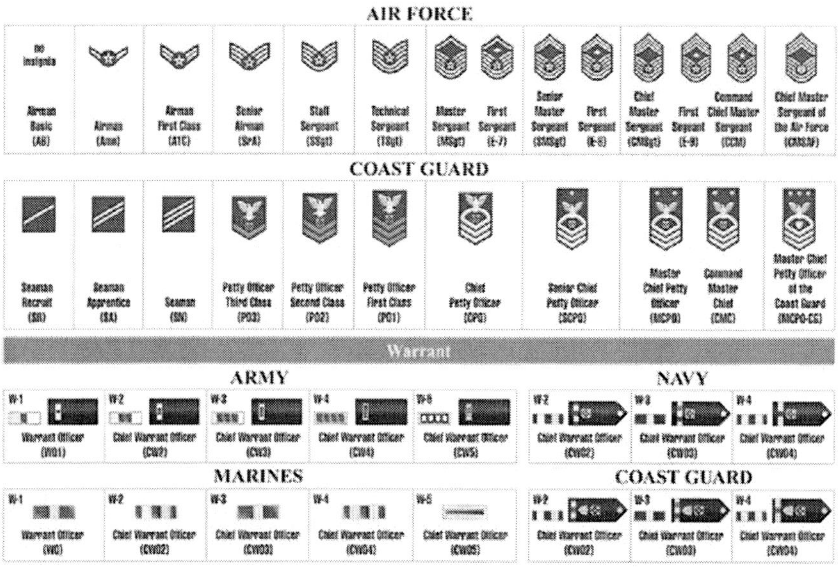

End Notes

[1] http://odam.defense.gov/omp/pubs/GuideBook/DoD.htm.

[2] Ibid.

[3] http://en.wikipedia.org/wiki/us armed forces#budget.

[4] 10 U.S.C. § 10102: Purpose of reserve components.

[5] "National Guard Deployments: Fact Sheet," CRS Report for Congress, January 17, 2008, http://www.fas.org/sgp/crs/natsec/RS22451.pdf.

[6] U.S. Army, Stand-To, June 30, 2009, http://www.army.mil/standto/archive/2009/06/30/.

[7] The Army is the only service component that made this change from a strategic reserve to an operational force.

[8] Department of Defense, Statistical Information Analysis Division, Personnel and Military Casualty Statistics, http://siadapp.dmdc.osd.mil/personnel/MMIDHOME.HTM. Department of Defense, Statistical Information Analysis Division,

[9] Department of Defense, Statistical Information Analysis Division, Personnel and Military Casualty Statistics, http://siadapp.dmdc.osd.mil/personnel/MMIDHOME.HTM.

[10] Department of Defense, Statistical Information Analysis Division, Personnel and Military Casualty Statistics, http://siadapp.dmdc.osd.mil/personnel/MILITARY/history/hst1009.pdf..

[11] Military Personnel: Reporting Additional Servicemember Demographics Could Enhance Congressional Oversight (GAO Report to Congressional Requestors), September 2005, http://www.gao.gov/new.items/d05952.pdf.

[12] Ibid.

[13] http://www.defense.gov/landing/questions.aspx.

[14] Steven L. Meyers, "Women at Arms: Living and Fighting Alongside Men, and Fitting In," New York Times, August 16, 2009.

[15] Ibid.

[16] Office of the Under Secretary of Defense, Personnel and Readiness, Population Representation in the Military Services, Fiscal Year 2005, http://prhome.defense.gov/poprep2005/contents/contents.html.

[17] "Military Personnel: Reporting Additional Servicemember Demographics Could Enhance Congressional Oversight", Report to Congressional Requesters, September 2005. http://www.gao.gov/new.items/d05952.pdf

[18] Elizabeth M. Collins, "Kids Affected With Repeat Deployments," Military.com, October 13, 2009, http://www.military.com/news/article/army-news/kids-affected-with-repeatdeployments.html?col=1186032369115.

[19] Seth Robson, "Some Seek Mental Health Checks for Spouses of Multiple-Deployed Soldiers," Stars and Stripes, European Edition, July 5, 2009.

[20] "War's Silent Stress: The Family at Home," Blue Star Voices blog post, August 19, 2009, http://bluestarfamilies.wordpress.com/2009/08/19/wars-silent-stress-the-family-at-home/.

[21] Collins, 2009.

[22] Report on the Cycles of Deployment: An Analysis of Survey Reponses from April Through September, 2005. Survey conducted by and report compiled by the National Military Family Association. http://www.alaskapta.org/NMFACyclesofDeployment9.pdf. The Cycles of Deployment survey was completed by 1,592 active and reserve component service members from six of the seven uniformed services—Army, Navy, Air Force, Marine Corps, Coast Guard and Public Health Services. Seventy percent of the respondents offered comments and personal stories.

[23] Gregg Zoroya, "Military Divorces Edge Up as War Takes Its Toll," USA Today, November 27, 2009.

[24] As of March 30, 2010, 37,155 men and women have been injured, as compared to 5,411 deaths. Weekly casualty totals as reported by the Department of Defense, http://www.defense.gov/news/casualty.pdf.

INDEX

A

abuse, 83, 86, 89
access, 9, 14, 17, 20, 22, 23, 27, 35, 36, 39, 42, 48, 49, 78, 79, 83, 85, 86
accessions, 74, 75
adjustment, 83
adrenaline, 84, 87
adults, 77
advancement, 63
advocacy, 13, 21, 22, 30, 32
Afghanistan, viii, 2, 6, 19, 21, 30, 54, 56, 60, 61, 63, 64, 65, 72, 73, 83, 85
African Americans, 74, 75
age, 5, 6, 7, 67, 74, 77
agencies, 3, 11, 14, 15, 16, 31, 37, 39, 40, 46
aggression, 88
Air Force, 61, 67, 69, 70, 72, 95
alcohol use, 21
alienation, 91
anxiety, 10, 77, 78, 89
appropriations, 61
aptitude, 74
armed conflict, 65
armed forces, 7, 63, 94
arrest, 10, 30, 36
Asian Americans, 74
assault, 73, 74
assessment, 4, 20, 28, 31, 33, 34, 37, 42
assessment tools, 4, 20, 31, 34, 37, 42
atmosphere, 88
authority(s), 24, 60, 61, 67, 68, 69, 84, 89, 90
awareness, 25, 28, 29, 33, 81, 86

B

barriers, vii, 2, 4, 14, 18, 22, 27, 29, 34, 36, 38, 39, 41, 46, 47, 48, 56
base, 14, 62, 76, 78, 79, 81, 85, 86
benchmarks, 67
benefits, 9, 10, 11, 14, 19, 25, 27, 33, 36, 37, 38, 39, 40, 79
blindness, 85
blueprint, 23
Bosnia, 64
breakdown, 72

C

caffeine, 86, 87
career development, 91
case study(s), vii, 2, 4, 8, 29, 34, 35, 36, 38, 39, 40, 42, 43
central planning, 21
chain of command, 61, 67, 68, 70, 74, 90
challenges, 19, 65, 77, 78, 79, 83
chemical(s), 64, 87, 91
Chicago, 64

Chief of Staff, 77
childcare, 27, 42
children, 20, 31, 36, 38, 77, 78, 82
city(s), 50, 52, 73
clarity, 83, 90, 91
clients, 3, 9, 13, 15, 23, 33, 37, 39, 40, 41
clinical presentation, 10
clinical symptoms, 25
clusters, 87
Coast Guard, 17, 61, 67, 69, 70, 72, 95
cognitive abilities, 82
collaboration, 18, 22, 32, 35, 38, 39, 42
communication, 35, 40, 46, 78, 83, 90
community(s), 3, 9, 13, 23, 27, 28, 29, 38, 39, 40, 41, 42, 62, 63, 64, 66, 76, 83, 89, 90, 92
community service, 42
community support, 90
community-based services, 39
compensation, 9
complement, 4, 22
concussion, 87
conference, 20, 25, 28
Conference Report, 54
conflict, 65
Congress, 60, 94
Constitution, 60, 63, 64
cooking, 66
coordination, 30, 35, 40
cost, 3, 18, 41, 42, 61
counseling, 11, 14, 30, 40
covering, 9
criminal justice system, 23
CT, 9, 46
culture, vii, viii, 2, 15, 16, 34, 37, 42, 59, 60, 66, 68, 70, 84, 86, 88, 89, 90
curricula, 4
cycles, 62, 87

D

danger, 38, 48, 73
data collection, 8, 12
database, 12
deaths, 63, 95
decision makers, 84
decision-making process, 69, 87
deficiencies, 87, 91
Department of Defense, 3, 23, 30, 61, 83, 86, 94, 95
Department of Homeland Security, 61
deployment(s), viii, 2, 17, 29, 36, 56, 60, 62, 64, 65, 76, 77, 78, 79, 82, 83, 89, 90
depression, 77, 78, 82
destruction, 80
differential diagnosis, 87
disability, 9
disappointment, 82
discharges, 15
discomfort, 91
disorder, vii, 2, 5, 33, 47, 48
District of Columbia, 63
diversity, 43
domestic violence, 37
draft, 23, 71
drugs, 14, 65, 86, 87

E

education, 8, 9, 10, 11, 21, 22, 26, 67, 75, 86, 90
educational materials, 29
eligibility criteria, 9
emergency, 27, 37, 64
emotion, 76
emotional health, 26
emotional reactions, 89
employees, 23, 25
employers, 10, 24, 27, 32, 65
employment, 65, 84, 90
enemies, 69
enrollment, 9
environment, 68, 71, 81
equipment, 65, 66, 67, 80, 85
ethics, 70, 74
evidence, 34, 36, 41
evidence-based practices, 34, 37, 41
exclusion, 72
execution, 61
executive function(s), 88

exercise, 87
expertise, 22
exposure, 28, 60

F

family members, vii, 1, 8, 9, 11, 14, 15, 24, 26, 30, 34, 35, 43, 46, 47, 49, 76, 77, 78, 79, 83, 84, 89, 90, 92
family support, 78, 90
family therapy, 90
fear, 35, 60, 73, 74, 79, 81
feelings, 91
fiber, 81
fidelity, 83, 88
fights, 69
financial, 20, 22, 27, 33, 38, 40, 42, 82
financial planning, 27, 33, 42
fires, 64
fiscal year 2009, 83
floods, 64
food, 62, 67, 80
force, viii, 17, 18, 19, 20, 23, 24, 27, 29, 39, 59, 62, 63, 65, 71, 74, 77, 94
forest fire, 64
funding, 8, 9, 11, 14, 16, 19, 21, 25, 27, 35, 38, 39, 48, 61
funds, 11, 13, 14, 21, 25, 28, 46, 47, 48

G

GAO, 94
geography, 19, 80
God, 80
governor, 17
grades, 66
growth, 92
guidance, 82
guilt, 81, 87, 88
Gulf Coast, 64

H

hair, 62
hand-to-hand combat, 71
harassment, 73, 74
healing, 89, 92
health, 2, 9, 11, 16, 17, 18, 19, 21, 23, 24, 27, 28, 29, 36, 38, 56, 64, 65, 66, 78, 84, 85
health care, 18, 23, 27, 56, 78
health care system, 18, 27
health insurance, 23, 38
health services, 9, 11, 19, 24, 27, 85
high school, 75
high school diploma, 75
Hispanics, 75
history, 60, 70, 94
honesty, 83
host, 28, 32
House, 17, 24
housing, 16, 23, 27, 32, 33, 40, 42, 76
human, viii, 59, 63, 64, 87
Hurricane Katrina, 64
husband, 82

I

identification, 23
immune function, 86
improvements, 19, 85
Indians, 74, 75
individuals, 12, 15, 18, 35, 41, 62, 63, 67, 74, 84, 86, 88, 92
injuries, 27, 28, 57, 82, 85
integration, 28
integrity, 68, 69, 92
intelligence, 80
interagency coordination, 3
intervention, 11, 19, 21, 90
intimacy, 82
Iraq, viii, 2, 6, 19, 21, 30, 54, 55, 56, 59, 61, 63, 64, 65, 72, 73, 82, 83, 85
Iraq War, 55
isolation, 66, 90
issues, 9, 10, 19, 22, 25, 26, 33, 34, 35, 37, 65, 78, 83, 85, 87, 88, 89

K

kill, 70, 71
Kosovo, 64

L

labeling, 12
law enforcement, vii, 2, 19, 26, 37, 42, 43, 64
lead, 46, 83
leadership, 35, 39, 66, 79
learning, 19, 47, 70, 92
legislation, 5, 10
lifetime, 76
living arrangements, 73
local authorities, 24
low risk, 26

M

majority, 70, 79
man, 67, 69
management, 11, 21, 23, 63, 86, 92
Marine Corps, 61, 66, 67, 69, 72, 95
marriage, 82, 83, 90
married couples, 73
materials, vii, 2, 17, 26, 34, 42, 46
matrix, 85
media, 77
medical, 14, 22, 27, 37, 70, 73, 85
medical care, 73, 85
medication, 86
mental health, 3, 8, 11, 12, 17, 18, 19, 20, 22, 23, 24, 25, 26, 27, 28, 37, 40, 42, 56, 64, 65, 77, 78, 85
mental illness, 23
Mexico, 4, 11, 12, 13, 30, 35, 36, 37, 38, 39, 40, 41, 44, 49
military conflicts, viii, 60
military occupation, 72
military personnel, viii, 8, 60, 70
military service, viii, 59, 60, 61, 69, 71, 80, 85, 88
minorities, 74, 75
mission(s), 61, 63, 64, 65, 66, 67, 69, 70, 71, 73, 80, 81, 84, 90, 91
models, vii, 2
musculoskeletal, 86

N

National Defense Authorization Act, 72
national emergency, 63
national security, 63
National Survey, 7
natural disaster, 64
negative consequences, 12
New England, 23, 24, 32, 56
nightmares, 82
NPS, 74, 75
nurses, 28

O

OCS, 70
officials, vii, 2, 37, 64
Operation Enduring Freedom, 2, 65
Operation Iraqi Freedom, 2, 65
operations, 57, 62, 64, 65, 66, 73
opportunities, 18, 77
optimization, 89
organize, 28
outpatient, 9, 16, 19
outreach, vii, 1, 3, 8, 9, 10, 11, 13, 14, 16, 18, 19, 20, 22, 24, 26, 27, 28, 29, 30, 31, 32, 37, 38, 40, 42, 47, 48, 78, 86
outreach efforts, vii, 2, 29, 42, 48
oversight, 21, 67
ownership, 63

P

Pacific, 74
Pacific Islanders, 74
pain, 65, 86, 87
pain management, 87
parents, 31, 36, 77

participants, 39, 47
peace, 61
Pentagon, 61
personal stories, 95
personality, 82
physicians, 14, 27, 28, 29, 33, 37, 38, 42
physiological factors, 91
pilot study, 12, 13
pleasure, 76
police, 11, 28, 64
policy, 4, 8, 9, 19, 30, 46, 61, 72, 73
policy initiative, 8, 46
policy issues, 9
policymakers, 12
population, 3, 5, 12, 14, 17, 19, 28, 34, 36, 37, 39, 41, 42, 43, 46, 74, 75, 80, 86
Posse Comitatus Act, 64
post traumatic stress disorder (PTSD), vii, 2
posttraumatic stress, 33
post-traumatic stress disorder, 74, 87
preparation, 36
President, 60, 61, 63, 64, 67
prevention, vii, 1, 2, 3, 11, 13, 14, 16, 21, 22, 26, 38, 39, 42, 46, 47, 48, 90
professionals, viii, 18, 22, 60, 85
programming, 39, 41
project, 9, 12, 13, 14, 23, 32
protection, 91
psychiatric disorders, 89
psychiatrist, 77
psychological problems, 74, 77
psychotropic medications, 86
PTSD, vii, 2, 10, 12, 16, 18, 20, 21, 22, 24, 25, 26, 27, 28, 29, 31, 32, 33, 34, 36, 37, 40, 42, 52, 55, 56, 74, 82, 87, 89
public service, 24, 32
pumps, 80

Q

qualifications, 62

R

radio, 29
reactions, 89
reality, 76, 80, 81
recommendations, vii, 2, 19, 42, 57, 68, 78
recovery, 3, 42
recruiting, 8, 16, 71
regulations, 67
rehabilitation, 9, 21
rehabilitation program, 9, 21
reimburse, 27
relaxation, 87
requirements, 9, 62, 65, 67
researchers, 83
reserves, 7, 9
Residential, 24
resilience, 81
resistance, 91
resources, vii, 1, 4, 8, 17, 20, 25, 27, 28, 30, 33, 34, 37, 39, 56, 66, 78, 79, 86, 91
response, 46, 47, 48, 64
restaurants, 62
restrictions, 10, 23
retaliation, 74
revenue, 41
rights, 64
risk(s), 2, 10, 30, 36, 56, 65, 68, 77, 81, 89
risk factors, 56
roots, 88, 89
rules, 67
rural areas, 18, 19

S

safety, 56, 68, 69, 74
SAMHSA, 2, 7, 9, 12, 14, 23, 36, 42, 49, 56
SAS, 17, 18
school, 14, 30, 38, 62, 64, 76, 77
scope, 5
Secretary of Defense, 61, 74, 95
security, 26, 35, 61, 71, 73
self-worth, 84
Senate, 67, 77

September 11, 19
service provider, 13, 17, 18, 21, 29
services, vii, 1, 2, 3, 4, 8, 9, 11, 12, 13, 14, 16, 17, 18, 19, 20, 22, 23, 25, 26, 27, 28, 31, 33, 34, 35, 36, 38, 39, 40, 41, 42, 43, 45, 48, 49, 62, 66, 69, 70, 76, 77, 83, 85, 86, 89, 90, 95
sexual assaults, 73
sexual harassment, 73, 88
shortage, 78
signs, 25, 29
sleep deprivation, 80, 86, 87, 88
social services, 30
society, 28, 60, 91
socioeconomic status, 75
South Dakota, 54
specialists, viii, 60, 86
spending, 61
SSA, vii, 2, 5, 8, 13, 18, 19, 29, 30, 35, 36, 37, 39, 40, 42, 45, 46, 47
stability, 27, 40
staff members, 14, 23
staffing, 32
stakeholder analysis, 19
stakeholders, 4, 8, 45
state(s), 23, 26, 53, 63, 64, 81
state authorities, 64
state of emergency, 64
statistics, 18, 73, 74, 75
stigma, 12, 25, 35, 41, 89
strategic planning, 9
stress, vii, 2, 68, 70, 76, 78, 80, 83, 87, 88, 89, 91, 92, 95
stressors, 78
structure, 10, 66, 79, 82, 84, 90, 91
substance abuse, 56
substance use, vii, 1, 2, 5, 7, 9, 11, 12, 13, 14, 15, 16, 17, 18, 19, 20, 22, 23, 24, 25, 26, 27, 28, 30, 31, 34, 35, 36, 37, 38, 39, 40, 41, 42, 43, 46, 47, 48, 64, 85, 86, 89, 91
Substance use disorder(s), vii, 1, 15, 48, 91
substitutes, 86
SUD, v, vii, 1, 2, 3, 8, 13, 16, 18, 20, 22, 31, 36, 37, 38, 39, 40, 41, 42, 43, 45
suicide, 77
suicide rate, 77
supervisor, 68
Supreme Court, 64
survival, 88
sustainability, 9
symptoms, 2, 10, 25, 26, 28, 36, 87, 91, 92
syndrome, 87

T

target, 19, 28, 29, 34, 36
target population(s), 29, 34
Task Force, 19, 20, 21, 22, 23, 24, 32, 52
TBI, vii, 2, 3, 10, 15, 16, 17, 18, 20, 26, 27, 28, 29, 30, 31, 33, 34, 36, 37, 40, 42, 82, 87
teachers, 10, 30
teams, 67
technical assistance, vii, 2, 3, 42
techniques, 87
technology, 28, 39, 41
telehealth, vii, 2, 12, 18, 28, 39, 41, 42
telephone, 17, 26, 27
telephone numbers, 26
tempo, 65, 77
tension, 86
territory, 63, 81
terrorism, 36
therapeutic process, 89, 91
therapeutic relationship, 91
therapist, 91
therapy, 89, 90, 91
thoughts, 88, 89
tracks, 4, 28
training, vii, 1, 3, 4, 8, 9, 10, 11, 13, 15, 16, 18, 20, 21, 22, 23, 24, 27, 28, 32, 33, 34, 35, 37, 39, 42, 43, 47, 61, 62, 63, 70, 71, 81, 84, 85, 89
training programs, 20, 28
transportation, vii, 2, 12, 23, 27, 33, 38, 39, 41, 42
trauma, vii, 2, 20, 23, 36, 37, 42, 56, 74, 85, 88
traumatic brain injury, vii, 2, 33, 82, 87

traumatic events, 38
treatment, vii, 1, 2, 3, 4, 5, 6, 7, 10, 12, 13, 14, 15, 16, 18, 19, 20, 21, 22, 25, 27, 28, 31, 35, 36, 37, 38, 39, 41, 42, 46, 47, 48, 56, 90

U

uniform, 62, 68, 70, 71, 84
uninsured, 19
United, 17, 60, 61, 66, 69, 72, 77, 92, 93
United States, 17, 60, 61, 66, 69, 72, 77, 92, 93
universe, 5
urban, 43
urban areas, 43
USA, 95

V

vehicles, 73, 80
venue, 20
Vice President, 14, 17
Vietnam, 71
violence, 26
vouchers, 12, 23
vulnerability, 86

W

waiver, 16
walking, 82, 87
war, 27, 28, 36, 57, 60, 61, 63, 64, 80, 81, 82, 86, 89
War on Terror, 17, 31
Washington, 77
water, 80
weapons, 71, 80
wear, 62, 70
web, 20, 31, 32, 39, 40, 41
webinar, vii, 2, 28, 41, 42
websites, 29
well-being, 66, 74, 84, 89
Wisconsin, 54
workers, vii, 2, 19, 37
workforce, 3, 23, 42, 43, 62, 66, 72, 74, 75
World War I, 34, 36, 65, 81
worry, 78, 90